Health Services Marketing
A Practitioner's Guide

D0993018

Richard K. Thomas

Health Services Marketing

A Practitioner's Guide

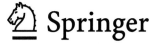 Springer

Richard K. Thomas
Health Management Associates
Memphis, TN
USA

ISBN-13: 978-0-387-73604-4   e-ISBN-13: 978-0-387-73606-8

Library of Congress Control Number: 2007934986

Printed on acid-free paper.

9 8 7 6 5 4 3 2 1

springer.com

Preface

The formal recognition in the 1980s of marketing as an appropriate activity for health services providers represented an important milestone. It led to the establishment of marketing budgets and the creation of numerous new positions within healthcare organizations, culminating with the establishment of the position of vice president for marketing in many organizations. This development opened healthcare up to an influx of concepts and methods from other industries and helped to introduce modern business practices into the healthcare arena.

The importance of marketing in healthcare today is reflected by the fact that many health professionals (*outside* the marketing department) are encouraged if not commanded to become marketers of a sort. Today, thousands of health professionals with no marketing background are being asked to develop marketing plans for their units. Even for those in healthcare who are not directly involved in marketing, there is likely to be a need at some point to interface with those who are.

This book is intended to provide an overall understanding of what marketing is – and isn't. It presents the basic concepts of marketing for the benefit of all likely to be faced with marketing challenges and describes the techniques that can be used to implement a marketing initiative. The book is intended to provide some of the basic skills – supported by ample resources – to lay the groundwork for developing a marketing plan and actually implementing a marketing campaign. Although one book is not likely to make the reader an expert on marketing, it is hoped that it provides enough information to establish a marketing mindset and set the process in motion.

Given the intent of this book, limited attention is paid to the history of healthcare marketing or to the theories that underlie this endeavor. The emphasis is on the nuts-and-bolts of marketing, with careful attention paid to the specific steps that must be taken to develop and implement a marketing plan. The long experience of the author yields numerous "tricks of the trade" that will facilitate the learning of marketing techniques. More than anything, this book is intended to be a "how-to" guide, supplemented by checklists, sample forms, questionnaires, and other materials that will facilitate the marketing process.

Ultimately, there are no marketing silver bullets. Since no one is born a marketing professional, we have to learn what works. Every organization is different, and we have to determine what works for each one. Since every market is also different you have to learn what works in your market vis-á-vis the competition. This book will not provide all of the answers but, hopefully, will tell you where to find them.

Given that virtually every development that's occurring in healthcare is pointing toward the need for more marketing, the demand for marketing skills is certainly going to grow. The payoff for the healthcare practitioner who understands marketing can be significant, and virtually every healthcare organization can be expected to increasingly value those skills.

Contents

Chapter 1
Introduction to Healthcare Marketing

Chapter 1 provides an introduction to marketing for health professionals. Although marketing has a long history in other industries, it is a relatively recent phenomenon in healthcare. In this chapter the case for marketing is made and what marketing can and can't do is discussed. The chapter offers guidance on who should do marketing and when they should do it.

What Marketing Is and Isn't

"Marketing," according to the American Marketing Association, is the process of planning and executing the conception, pricing, promotion, and distribution of ideas, goods, and services to create exchanges that satisfy individual and organizational objectives. "Healthcare marketing" extends this definition of marketing to the healthcare field. Viewed broadly, healthcare marketing involves any activities that relate to the development, packaging, pricing and distribution of healthcare products and to any mechanisms used for promoting these products.

It should be noted that marketing is not just advertising or public relations or direct mail or any number of other promotional techniques that might be utilized. Marketing is not embodied by any one technique, but they are all part of the marketing process, and should all be used within the context of the institution's marketing plan. All too often in healthcare the term marketing is used to reference one of these specific functions, masking the range of activities carried out under the umbrella of marketing and the extent to which marketing should pervade the organization. As will be seen, marketing is a broad endeavor that involves a wide range of activities.

Why Marketing is the Hardest Job in Healthcare

Despite the growing acceptance of marketing, healthcare marketers continue to face numerous challenges. They will find that few healthcare administrators have been trained in the business aspects of healthcare, and fewer still have had training in or experience with marketing. Many in healthcare even continue to be skeptical about the appropriateness of marketing. For some health professionals, business practices still carry an unfavorable connotation that implies the subjugation of clinical concerns to the bottom line. There are even some lingering industry restrictions on marketing that discourage or outright prohibit certain marketing activities.

Even among those health professionals that are accepting of marketing, there is concern over the return on investment (ROI) that marketing can generate. Even today, healthcare organizations are seldom able to measure the cost of providing a specific service, making cost/benefit analyses extremely difficult.

Marketers seldom get the recognition they deserve from health professionals and their efforts are likely to go unnoted and unrewarded. Marketing is still considered to be a "necessary evil" by some, and, to them, putting up with marketers is a price that has to be paid to compete in the modern world.

Finally, healthcare marketers may not have access to the resources and capabilities that they are used to in other industries. Box 1.1 indicates some of the "deficiencies" that exist in healthcare from the point of view of the marketer.

Why Marketing is the Best Job in Healthcare

The changing healthcare environment has brought marketing front and center. Most of the trends affecting healthcare point to the need for increased marketing involvement, and all of the current developments in healthcare have a marketing dimension. As more interface is required between healthcare organizations and their environments, the role of the marketer will only grow in importance. More and more, marketing is becoming the "action end" of healthcare.

Healthcare is a dynamic industry that requires creativity and passion of its marketers. Healthcare marketing is still in its early stages of development and, as such, is characterized by an air of excitement and exploration. Not only are new products and services constantly being introduced, but the fact that there are few established marketing procedures in healthcare makes for an exciting environment. There is little that is routine about healthcare marketing, and numerous opportunities exist in this fluid environment that might not be found in other, more established industries.

Box 1.1 What the marketer shouldn't expect in healthcare

Marketers entering healthcare from other fields may be surprised to find that they do not necessarily have the same resources and capabilities that they previously had. Part of this is due to the newness of marketing in healthcare and part due to the unique characteristics of the Industry. Examples of "gaps" in resources that the healthcare marketer might encounter are outlined below.

Standardized marketing techniques – There is little in healthcare marketing that is standardized and much of it has to be made up as we go. Marketing techniques cannot necessarily be adopted from other fields and few "routine" marketing approaches have been established.

Industry data – In most industries the various entities cooperate to establish clearinghouses of information for use by all industry interests. This is generally not the case in healthcare due to the fragmentation of the system, the local nature of healthcare services and restrictions that are placed on the use of patient data.

Well-defined products – Health professionals are not used to thinking in terms of "products" so little thought has been given to the definition and packaging of the services provided by healthcare organizations. Marketers often must redefine amorphous services as products for promotional purposes.

Routine resources – Marketers might expect to have access to support staff, advertising budgets, research funds and a variety of other resources that are prerequisites for a marketing department. These resources may not be in place in the typical healthcare organization and the marketer may find himself starting from scratch to to meet even basic needs.

Customer profiles – Because of the lack of industry data, the marketer may be faced with a paucity of data on the target audiences of the organization. Because of the importance of referral networks and health plan steering, many healthcare organizations have not emphasized the characteristics of their customers, a deficiency reinforced by restrictions placed on the use of patient data.

Clear outcome measures – The effectiveness of most marketing initiatives can be easily assessed using standard evaluation techniques. This is not the case in healthcare where the results of a marketing initiative might be measured in different ways, and the actual impact of marketing (vis-à-vis other activities) may be hard to discern.

Appreciation – Since marketing remains a "necessary evil" for many in healthcare, it is not surprising that healthcare marketers are not universally loved and adored. Rather than recognizing the positive contributions made by marketing, health professionals might perceive of marketers as a distraction from the true mission of the organization and a competitor for scarce resources.

Who Should Market?

The question of "who should market" can be addressed at a couple of different levels (although the real question in today's healthcare environment should be: "Who *shouldn't* market?"). When we talk about Marketing (with a capital "M") it can be argued that every healthcare organization needs to be involved in marketing in one form or another. We often associate marketing with large organizations like hospitals and health systems with their substantial advertising budgets. Yet, it is not the size of the organization that determines the need for marketing, it is the nature of the environment in which it operates. And today's healthcare environment has become increasingly competitive. The mom-and-pop home health agency needs to market as much as a large national chain although the approach might be quite different. Even monopolistic organizations realize that they have to market to maintain customer satisfaction and assure high morale among their employees.

When we consider marketing (with a little "m") we might consider the need for everyone in the organization to be something of a marketer. In a true "marketing organization" everyone should be considered a "salesperson" for the organization and, as such, they need to be familiar with marketing concepts. At the same time, managers with no marketing background are increasingly being asked to develop marketing plans for their departments or units. Indeed, the ability to continue to obtain resources for their department may depend on the existence of a sound marketing plan.

Why Healthcare is Different

Healthcare is different from other industries in many ways that have implications for marketing. In other industries, there is an assumption that buyers are driven primarily, if not exclusively, by economic motives. This assumption often does not hold in healthcare. In fact, a number of factors operate to prevent the buyers of health services from operating in the same manner as the buyers of lawn services or accounting services.

The existence of a market also assumes that there is a competitive situation in which sellers compete for the consumer's resources and that this competition determines the price of the goods and services offered. In healthcare, however, it is not unusual for one or a small number of healthcare providers to maintain control over a particular service within a particular market. For this reason, healthcare costs may not be influenced by the laws of supply and demand.

Because of the unusual financing arrangement characterizing healthcare, healthcare consumers seldom know the price of the services they are consuming until after they have consumed them. In fact, the physician or clinician providing the service may not even know the price of the service being provided. Since the end-user is seldom required to pay directly for the service consumed – this is left up to third-party payers in the typical case – they may not even notice how much their care costs.

Healthcare organizations have numerous characteristics that have implications for marketing. For example, healthcare organizations tend to be multipurpose activities, and large organizations like hospitals are likely to pursue a number of goals simultaneously. Indeed, an academic medical center may emphasize education, research, or community service with patient care being a secondary function. Even large specialty practices may have a more diffuse orientation than organizations in other industries.

Most healthcare organizations are chartered as not-for-profit organizations. This not-for-profit orientation creates an environment that is much different from that characterizing other industries. Marketers coming from other industries may be surprised to find that healthcare organizations often willingly provide services that are not likely to turn a profit. The fact that many health facilities and programs operate with government support also creates a different dynamic.

When healthcare organizations may provide services that are not profitable, it may reflect the fact that certain services (e.g., emergency rooms at hospitals) are legally mandated to accept any presenting patient; in others, it reflects the fact that hospitals, and to a lesser degree physicians, must offer the comprehensive services required by the community in order to remain competitive.

Except for elective procedures for which the consumer pays out of pocket, most of the decisions that impact the demand for health services are made by gatekeepers such as physicians and health plans. The end-user may have little or nothing to say with regard to decisions related to care, and the marketer may have to reach the end-user indirectly through some intermediary.

Healthcare organizations are also unique in the emphasis placed on referral relationships. Hospitals depend on admissions from their medical staffs, and their staff members in turn depend on referrals from other physicians. Indeed, except in emergency situations, patients can only gain hospital admission through a referral. Many specialists will not accept self-referred patients and rely on other physicians for their customers. The same types of referral relationships exist with regard to other services (e.g., home healthcare, nursing homes). Marketing to the end-user may not be effective when referral relationships are important.

The role that health plans play in channeling customers to various providers can not be overlooked. Health plans may require patients to utilize particular providers or facilities and may even insist on authorizing any such referrals. In no other industry do parties who are not the end-user exert such an influence on the process.

Marketers are understandably interested in the nature of the products (most often services) offered by healthcare organizations. After all, this is what is going to be marketed. While many healthcare consumer goods (e.g., band-aids, fitness equipment, and over-the-counter drugs) may be marketed just as any other product, most healthcare products do not fall into this category. Indeed, even the most common of consumer-oriented healthcare products – pharmaceuticals – must be prescribed by a middleman before they can be acquired and consumed.

Healthcare providers are generally concerned with the promotion of a service that is often difficult to describe. The things that providers are likely to think they provide (e.g., quality care, prolongation of life, elimination of pathology) are often hard to define or measure. The difficulty in specifying the services provided becomes obvious to the marketer who asks a hospital department head what services the department provides.

Few services stand alone but often come in "bundles" (e.g., the group of services that surrounds a particular surgical procedure). While clinicians (and their billing clerks) may see them as discrete services, the patient perceives them as a complex mix of services related to a traumatic event, diabetes management or cancer treatment.

The healthcare industry has been historically dominated by "professionals" rather than by businessmen. Clinical personnel (usually physicians, but other clinicians as well) define much of the demand for health services and are responsible directly or indirectly for the majority of healthcare expenditures. Yet these clinicians may not have the same goals and objectives as administrators. The medical ethics that drive the behavior of health professionals exists independently of the operation of the system. Decisions made in the best medical interests of the patient may not be the most profitable for the organization.

"Consumers" refers to those individuals with the potential to consume a particular good or service. Virtually everyone is likely to utilize healthcare goods or services at some time. The majority of the population visits a physician at least once during the year, and most of those who do use physician services report more than one visit. A large portion of the population is under pharmaceutical management, and virtually everyone purchases over-the-counter drugs at some point. This is not to mention those who purchase fitness equipment, self-help books, health food, and a variety of other "supportive" goods and services.

Another factor setting healthcare consumers apart from other consumers is the personal nature of the services involved. While few healthcare encounters involve matters of life or death, virtually all of them involve an emotional component that is absent in other consumer transactions. Every diagnostic test is fraught with the possibility of a "positive" result, and every surgery, no matter how minor, carries the potential for complications. Today's well-informed consumers are aware of the level of medical errors characterizing hospital care and the amount of system-induced morbidity associated with healthcare settings. Whether this emotionally charged and personal aspect of the healthcare episode prevents the affected individual from seeking care, colors the choice of provider or therapy, or leads to additional symptoms, the choices made by the patient or other decision makers are likely to be affected. Emotions like fear, pride and vanity often come into play more so than with the purchase of other goods and services.

Why Healthcare Marketing is Different

After considering the barriers to healthcare marketing outlined above, it becomes obvious that, to the extent that marketing does exist in healthcare, it is going to be different from marketing in other contexts. As many marketers from other industries have found out, marketing philosophies and techniques cannot readily be transferred from other contexts to healthcare. For this reason, healthcare requires its own unique approach and takes on certain characteristics unlike those of other industries.

One factor that makes healthcare marketing different is the nature of the demand for health services. While there is a certain elasticity in the demand for health services overall and there are elective procedures for which demand can actually be generated, most major healthcare episodes occur relatively rarely and almost always unpredictably. Such major events as a heart attack, a stroke or the onset of cancer are likely to arise unexpectedly and affect a small segment of the population. The marketing of such services represents a particular challenge for marketers who are faced with a disconnect between the service and the anticipated need.

Second, the end-user may not be the target for the marketing campaign. In virtually every other industry, the end user is responsible for the purchase decision and the decision maker actually consumes the good or service. This is often not the case in healthcare where a physician is likely to determine the what, where, when and how much of the service that is to be provided. The decision maker may be a physician, a health plan representative, a family member or some party other than the one who eventually consumes the service. The marketer is faced with the challenge of determining where to place the promotional emphasis under these circumstances.

Healthcare is also different in that the product may be highly complex and not lend itself to easy conceptualization. Many healthcare procedures, especially those that rely on technology, are complicated and difficult to explain to a layperson. Marketing such procedures to an audience that is already somewhat intimidated by the status of the physician and his medical jargon represents a particular challenge.

Another challenge peculiar to healthcare, particularly in the case of healthcare providers, is the situation where not all potential customers for a particular health service are considered "desirable." While healthcare providers are bound to a certain extent to provide services to anyone who presents with a problem regardless of their ability to pay, there are certain categories of patients that the marketer might not want to encourage to appear for services. For example, there may be cases where the Medicaid program reimburses at a very low rate for a particular service. Or there may be services where individuals without insurance (or other resources) are likely to present themselves for care. The marketer is faced with the challenge of attracting customers to the healthcare organization without over-attracting those who are likely to represent economic liabilities.

It is difficult to differentiate between healthcare providers that offer similar services. This is particularly true with hospitals and physician groups. Information may not be available that would allow quantitative comparisons between organizations and, even when it is available (e.g., comparative hospital pricing), it may not be very meaningful due to varying approaches in calculating patient fees. When all organizations have comparable attributes, it is difficult to make a case for a comparative advantage of one over the other.

Healthcare marketing, to a great extent, shares a problem with certain other industries and that is the challenge of marketing services rather than goods. For our purposes, "products" can be either "goods" or "services." Relative to goods, services are intangible and much more difficult to conceptualize. The purchase of goods tends to be a one-shot process, while services may be on going. It is more difficult to quantify services, and consumers evaluate them differently from more tangible products. Since services are often more "personal" (especially in the case of healthcare), they are likely to be assessed in subjective rather than objective terms.

Justifications for Healthcare Marketing

By the late 1970s, the arguments against investing in healthcare marketing were being stripped away one by one. While marketing was still a long way from being enthusiastically embraced, the reasons *for* incorporating marketing as a corporate function were beginning to mount up. The following justifications began to be put forth to support marketing efforts during this period:

Building awareness. With the introduction of new products and the emergence of an informed consumer, healthcare organizations were required to build awareness of their services and expose target audiences to their capabilities.

Enhancing visibility or image. With the increasing standardization of healthcare services and a growing appreciation of "reputation," healthcare organizations found it necessary to initiate marketing campaigns that would improve top-of-mind awareness and distinguish them from their competitors.

Improving market penetration. Healthcare organizations were faced with growing competition, and marketing represented a means for increasing patient volumes, growing revenues, and gaining market share. With few new patients in many markets, marketing was critical for retaining existing customers and attracting customers from competitors.

Increasing prestige. For many healthcare organizations, especially hospitals, it was felt that success hinged on being able to surpass competitors in terms of prestige. If prestige could be gained through having the best doctors, latest equipment and nicest facilities, these factors needed to be conveyed to the general public.

Attracting medical staff and employees. As the healthcare industry expanded, competition for skilled workers increased. Hospitals and other healthcare providers found it necessary to promote themselves to potential employees by marketing the superior benefits that they offered to recruits. With today's shortages of various health professionals, the ability to effectively market to prospective employees is critical.

Serving as an information resource. As healthcare became more complex and healthcare organizations offered a growing array of services, these organizations needed to constantly inform the general public and the medical community about the products they had to offer. Whether through press releases or recorded telephonic announcements, there was growing pressure to "get the word out."

Influencing consumer decision making. Once it was realized that the consumer had a role to play in healthcare decision making, the role of marketing in influencing this process was recognized. Whether it involved convincing consumers to decide on a particular organization's services or to speed up the decision-making process, marketing was becoming increasingly important.

Offsetting competitive marketing. Once healthcare organizations realized that their competitors were adopting aggressive marketing approaches, they began to adopt a stance of defensive marketing. They felt compelled to respond to the gambits of competitors by "out-marketing" them. This should not ever be the most important reason for marketing, but it would be unwise to ignore the marketing efforts of competitors.

(Box 1.2 indicates some myths that have affected the role of marketing in healthcare.)

Box 1.2 Eight marketing myths

Although healthcare marketing has made significant strides as a profession in recent years, the industry continues to struggle with the appropriate role for marketing at the corporate level. As one hospital administrator put it: "Healthcare marketing is like a chameleon trying to walk on hot rocks. Not only must it dance, but it most constantly change its appearance."

In actuality the profession has matured greatly since the 1980s, becoming more of a science and less of an art and finding ways to demonstrate its effectiveness to even its most vitriolic critics. Despite these advances, the full potential of marketing is often not reached because many in healthcare continue to harbor myths about marketing. Some of these myths are presented below, along with the actual facts.

Myth 1: Marketing doesn't matter.
Fact: It may be better to say that marketing cannot change everything. Admittedly, there are some things that marketing cannot change but, even there, marketing can serve to explain, clarify and justify those situations. *Efffective* marketing matters a lot.

Myth 2: Marketing equals advertising.
Fact: All advertising is marketing but not all marketing is advertising. Marketing aligns strategy with goals and objectives and establishes the framework for promotional activities. Advertising represents a tactic and *a* form of promotion among the many choices available to the marketer.

Myth 3: Consumers rule in healthcare.
Fact: Consumers may be more important in healthcare today than in the past but, more often than not, they must be cultivated through indirect means. The best way to reach the consumer is through relationships with physicians, health plans, and other organizations serving the consumer. Consumers *are, however,* becoming better at recognizing effective healthcare and are likely to respond accordingly.

Myth 4: The size of the marketing budget determines success.
Fact: Big budgets make marketers happy but unless the money is spent effectively much of it may be wasted. Uniqueness in the marketplace combined with credibility and consistency are the three wise kings of healthcare marketing. Ultimately, how *well* the marketing budget is used is more important than its size.

(continued)

Box 1.2 (continued)

Myth 5: Public relations is not important.
Fact: Public relations is a fundamental component of the promotional mix. PR can take advantage of current events, timing and marketing flexibility. The brand of an institution lives in the mind of consumers who evaluates your organization based on what they hear, believe and remember. Public relations has the advantage of receiving third-party endorsement by coming from the media.

Myth 6: Clever names and logos sell healthcare.
Fact: Clever product names and logos might attract attention, but unless they are part of an overall package of services associated with the parent institution they may well compete with your institution's position in the market. The situation is analogous to a family reunion where the individuals are secondary to the family.

Myth 7: Creativity drives the message.
Fact: People who judge marketing in terms of its creativity are typically not those consuming the services. Being creative for the sake of creativity only presents the illusion of marketing. Credibility, appropriate levels of reach and frequency, and competitive uniqueness have broader impact. If flashy marketing garners awards and not customers, the effort is wasted.

Myth 8: Marketing fads generate new business.
Fact: While it may be tempting to capitalize on the current fad, consistency really is king. The mind of the consumer is slower to hear than we are to speak. Their minds are even slower to believe what we say, and still slower to remember it. Using an "ad of the month" approach without a consistent position for the institution is likely to result in a poor return on your marketing investment.

Source: Used with permission from Thomas, Richard K., and Michael Calhoun (2007). *Marketing Matters: A Guide for Healthcare Executives*. Chicago: Health Administration Press, pp. 14–16.

Chapter 2
The Basics of Marketing

Chapter 2 introduces the basic marketing concepts that are utilized in healthcare and other industries. For those who are new to healthcare marketing, this will provide an introduction to the basics. For those with marketing experience, this section will reframe marketing concepts within the healthcare context. Marketing veterans will find the discussion of these concepts useful in explaining these concepts to health professionals with little experience with marketing.

Basic Concepts

Marketing

As noted earlier, marketing is the process of planning and executing the conception, pricing, promotion, and distribution of ideas, goods, and services to create exchanges that satisfy individual and organizational objective. "Healthcare marketing" would be defined by extending the initial definition of marketing to the healthcare field.

A parsing of the definition of marketing provides some important information about this endeavor. First, marketing involves a *process*, implying that the marketing operation involves a well thought out and systematic approach. The inclusion of *planning* in the definition indicates that marketing should not be done impulsively. The definition refers to four *components* of the marketing process (elsewhere referred to as the four Ps), to include product conception, pricing, promotion, and distribution channels (or the "place") through which the products are distributed.

Ultimately, the intent of marketing is to meet the goals of the organization (as seller) while, at the same time, meeting the goals of the customer (as buyer). Unless the goals of both parties are met, the marketing process would be considered unsuccessful. The challenge for the marketer is to identify the respective goals of buyers and sellers and facilitate mutually beneficial goal achievement, all within the context of establishing and enhancing the organization's reputation.

Marketing Planning

"Marketing planning" may be defined as the development of a systematic process for promoting an organization, a service or a product. This straightforward definition masks the wide variety of activities and potential complexity that characterize marketing planning. Marketing planning can be used address a short-term promotional project or comprise a component of a long-term strategic plan. It can focus alternatively on a product, service, program, or organization. Regardless of the focus, the plan serves as a guideline for all those involved in the company's marketing activities.

Marketing plans are by definition market driven, and they are single-minded in their focus on the customer. Whether the targeted customer is the patient, the referring physician, the employer, the health plan, or any number of other possibilities, the marketing plan is built around someone's needs. Although a consideration of internal factors is often pertinent (and "internal marketing" may be a component of many marketing plans), the marketing plan focuses on the characteristics of the external market with the objective of influencing change in one or more of these characteristics.

Marketing Management

"Marketing management" refers to the analysis, planning, implementation, and control of programs designed to achieve marketing objectives. The steps involved in the marketing management process include: (1) analyzing marketing opportunities, (2) selecting target markets, (3) developing the marketing mix, and (4) managing the marketing effort.

While marketing management is a well-defined function in most industries, it is still in its infancy in healthcare. The fragmented approach to much of the marketing that has taken place and the immature status of marketing in healthcare reflect the slow development of marketing management skills.

Marketing Research

"Marketing research" is the function that links the consumer, customer, and public to the marketer through information used to identify and define marketing opportunities and problems; generate, refine, and evaluate marketing actions; monitor marketing performance; and improve understanding of the marketing process. Often used interchangeably with "market research," marketing research is usually thought to encompass market research, product research, pricing research, promotional research, and distribution research. The marketing research process serves to identify the nature of the product or service, the characteristics of consumers, the size of the potential market, the nature of competitors, and any number of other essential pieces of the marketing puzzle.

Marketing Techniques

The activities that we generally think of as marketing actually represent only one component of the marketing process. The techniques that are used to promote an idea, organization or product must be viewed within the overall context. Marketing techniques range from the simple to the complex, from the inexpensive to the outrageously expensive. The arsenal of promotional options includes old standbys such as public relations and communications, approaches that predated the modern marketing era, along with "softer" approaches to promotions such as networking and community outreach.

More contemporary approaches include sales promotion, personal selling and direct mail. The wide range of activities that come under the heading of "advertising" are also options to be considered – from traditional advertising media (radio and newspapers) to more contemporary forms such as cable television and Internet marketing. Newer marketing techniques take advantage of contemporary technology, with database marketing, customer relationship management and direct-to-consumer marketing all relying on sophisticated information management capabilities.

"Levels" of Marketing

It is important to note that marketing can take place at a number of different "levels," measured primarily by the scope of the market being cultivated. For our purposes, these include mass marketing, target marketing and micromarketing.

Mass Marketing

"Mass marketing" refers to marketing efforts that involve the use of broad scope media that essentially target the entire market. Most frequently utilized by large national firms, mass marketing might utilize network television for the distribution of a consistent message to essentially the entire population. Mass marketing involves a one-size-fits-all message beamed indiscriminately into the market space. In the early days of healthcare marketing, healthcare organizations, particularly hospitals, typically used mass media to promote all services to all members of the target audience without regard for the fact that different segments of the audience might require different services.

Target Marketing

"Target marketing" refers to marketing initiatives that focus on a market segment to which an organization desires to offer goods/services. Target marketing stands in contrast to mass marketing in which the promotional efforts are aimed at the total market. While mass marketing involves a shotgun approach, target marketing is more of a rifle approach. Target markets in healthcare may be defined based on geography, demographics, lifestyles, insurance coverage, usage rates and/or other customer attributes. Thus, target marketing is likely to involve the use of some type of customer segmentation system.

Micromarketing

"Micromarketing" is a form of target marketing in which marketers tailor their promotions to the needs and wants of narrowly defined geographic, demographic, psychographic, or benefit segments. Customers and potential customers are identified at the household or individual level in order to promote goods and/or services directly to selected targets. Micromarketing is most effective when consumers with a narrow range of attributes must be reached.

The Nature of Healthcare Products

The definition of marketing offered early in this chapter refers to the promotion of ideas, goods or services. (The term "product," as will be seen throughout the text, is often used interchangeably with healthcare "service.") In contrast to other industries, it is often difficult to precisely specify the product that is to be marketed. Most of what is offered by healthcare organizations takes the form of services and, unlike goods, they tend to be more nebulous when it comes to description.

In addition, the nature of the product in healthcare has changed dramatically over the past couple of decades. Twenty years ago, one could define the product simply as a medical procedure, an orthotic device to correct a physical disability or a consumer health product. In today's climate, healthcare products include not only these traditional products, but also products and services such as prepaid health insurance plans offered by health maintenance organizations (HMOs) or a group purchasing contract offered by a provider network. (The nature of healthcare products is discussed further in Chapter 8.)

Many healthcare organizations offer a variety of products to their customers. Certainly, the hospital is an example of an organization that offers a wide range of services and goods. Indeed, a major hospital will offer hundreds if not thousands of different procedures. In addition, they offer a variety of goods (in the form of drugs doses, supplies and equipment) that are charged to the customer.

We can speak of an organization's product mix as it relates to the combination of services, goods and even ideas that it offers. Each of these concepts is addressed below.

Ideas

Much of what healthcare organizations promote takes the form of ideas or intangible concepts that are intended to convey a perception to the consumer. The organization's image is an idea that is likely to be conveyed through marketing activities. The organization may want to promote the perception of quality care, professionalism, value or some other subjective attribute. The intent, of course, is to establish a mindset that places the organization at the top of the consumer's mind on the assumption that familiarity will breed utilization.

When advertising was first adopted by healthcare organizations, most of the attention was accorded to the promotion of ideas. In particular, early marketers attempted to promote the organization's image and establish it as the preferred provider in its market. While the trend has been away from image advertising and toward service advertising, many healthcare organizations continue to market ideas to their target audiences.

Goods

A "good" refers to a tangible product that is typically purchased in an impersonal setting on a one-at-a-time basis. The purchase of goods tends to be a one-shot episode, while services may represent an on-going process. While we generally think of healthcare in terms of a service, the sale of goods is ubiquitous in the industry. Consumer health products (e.g., band-aids, condoms, toothpaste) are common household products. Pharmaceuticals – whether prescription or over-the-counter – are purchased by virtually everyone at some point. Home testing kits and therapeutic equipment are increasingly being acquired by consumers, and the sale and rental of durable medical equipment is a major industry. Even in a hospital setting, the bill for care is likely to include a number of goods among the itemized charges.

Services

Relative to goods, "services" are difficult to conceptualize. Services (e.g., physical examinations) are intangible in that they do not take on the concrete form of goods (e.g., drugs). It is more difficult to quantify services, and consumers evaluate them differently from more tangible products. Since services are often more "personal" (especially in the case of healthcare), they are likely to be assessed in subjective rather than objective terms. Services cannot be subjected to the quality controls placed on goods but reflect the variations that characterize the human beings who provide the services in a particular place at a particular time. Services are perishable in that they cannot be stored and once provided they have no residual value.

Healthcare Consumers and Other Target Audiences

A marketing activity must be directed to someone or something and a number of terms are used to refer to the target for marketing. After having answered the question "What are we marketing," the next question becomes "To whom are we marketing it?" Just as the healthcare "product" has been undergoing change, so has the healthcare "customer." While healthcare organizations not involved in patient care have long used business terminology for the customers, healthcare providers have more recently undergone redefinition of the party that uses their services. Producers of consumer health products have always had their "purchasers" and insurance plans their "members," but now the customer for healthcare providers is being transformed from a "patient" into a "consumer," "customer," "client," or some other manifestation that is more in keeping with the current healthcare environment. Some of the terms that are used for those consuming healthcare are defined below.

Consumers

"Consumer," as usually used in healthcare, refers to any individual or organization that is a potential purchaser of a healthcare product. (This differs from the more economics-based notion of consumer as the entity that actually *consumes* the product.) Theoretically, everyone is a potential consumer of health services, and consumer research, for example, is generally aimed at the public at large. The consumer is often the end-user of a good or service but may not necessarily be the purchaser. "Consumer behavior" refers to the utilization patterns and purchasing practices of the population of a market area.

Customers

The "customer" is typically thought of in healthcare as the actual purchaser of a good or service. While a patient may be a customer for certain goods and services, it is often the case that the end-user (i.e., the patient) may not be the customer. Someone else may make the purchase on behalf of the patient. Further, treatment decisions may be made by someone other than the patient.

For this reason, hospitals and other complex healthcare organizations are likely to serve a range of customers. These may include patients, referral agents, admitting physicians, employers, and a variety of other parties who may purchase goods or services from the organization. For this reason, the customer identification process in healthcare is more complicated than it is in other industries.

Clients

A "client" is a type of customer that consumes services rather than goods. A client relationship implies personal (rather than impersonal) interaction and an on-going relationship (rather than an episode). Professionals typically have clients while retailers, for example, have customers or purchasers. Clients are likely to have a more symmetrical relationship with the service provider than a patient who is typically dependent and powerless relative to the service provider. Many also feel that the term "client" implies more respect than the term "patient."

Patients

While the term "patient" is used rather loosely in informal discussion, a patient is technically someone who has been defined as sick by a physician. This almost always implies formal contact with a clinical facility (e.g., physician's office, hospital). Technically, a symptomatic individual does not become a patient until a physician officially designates the individual as such, even if he has consumed over-the-counter drugs and taken other measures for self-care. Under this scenario, an individual remains a patient until he is discharged from medical care.

While nonphysician clinicians may treat patients, it is often not considered appropriate for them to use that term. For example, mental health therapists are likely to refer to their patients as clients. Those dependent practitioners who work under the supervision of physicians (e.g., physical therapists), however, may define those who use their services as patients.

Enrollees

While health insurance plans have historically conceptualized their customers as "enrollees," this is a concept that has only recently become common among healthcare providers. However, with the ascendancy of managed care as a major force in healthcare, other healthcare organizations began to adopt this term. Thus, providers who contract to provide services for members of a health plan have begun to think in terms of enrollees. This is a significant shift in nomenclature, since an enrollee has different attributes from a patient. Enrollees may be variously referred to as members, insureds, or covered lives.

End-Users

End-users in health care, as in other industries, refers to the individuals who ultimately "consume" the product. In healthcare, that is generally the patient but could also be the purchaser of fitness equipment or a participant in a health education class. The situation in healthcare is complicated in that the end-user may not be the decision maker and, in fact, there may be any number of factors that cut the actual end-user out of the decision-making process. The end-user (often defined as a "consumer") is gaining increasing attention, however, in a more consumer-driven healthcare system. A current example of this would be the direct-to-consumer (read: end-user) marketing being carried out by many pharmaceutical companies.

The Four Ps of Marketing

The marketing mix is the set of controllable variables that an organization involved in marketing uses to influence the target market. The mix includes product, place, price, and promotion. The four Ps have long provided the framework for marketing strategy in other industries and are increasingly being considered by healthcare organizations. However, as will be seen, these aspects of the marketing mix do not necessarily have the same meaning for health professionals as they do for marketers in other contexts.

Product

The first "P," the "product" of healthcare, represents what healthcare organizations are marketing. The product represents the goods, services, or ideas offered by a healthcare organization. The product is sometimes difficult to precisely define in healthcare, and this creates a challenge for healthcare marketers.

"Products" can refer to either "goods" or "services." A good refers to a tangible product that is typically purchased in an impersonal setting on a one-at-a-time basis. Relative to goods, services are difficult to conceptualize. Services are intangible in that they do not take on the concrete form of goods. It is more difficult to quantify services, and consumers evaluate them differently from more tangible products.

Healthcare providers have seldom given much thought to the product concept in the past. Today, however, the design of the product, its perceived attributes, and its packaging are all becoming more important concerns for both healthcare providers and marketers.

Price

"Price" refers to the amount that is charged for a healthcare product. These include the fees, charges, premium contributions, deductibles, co-payments, and other out-of-pocket costs to consumers for health services. An employee paying an annual premium to a health plan, an insurance company reimbursing a physician's fee, or a consumer purchasing over-the-counter drugs all provide a product for a specified price.

The issue of pricing for health services is becoming a growing concern for marketers, and a number of factors are contributing to the greater role of the pricing variable in developing marketing strategy. For marketers, the challenge is in developing an understanding of what a customer is willing to exchange for some want-satisfying good or service and developing a pricing approach compatible with the goals of the organization and its cost constraints.

Place

The third "P", "place," represents the manner in which goods or services are distributed for use by consumers. Place might refer to the location or the hours a health service can be accessed. Increasingly, as more healthcare organizations establish relationships with managed care plans, the place variable assumes a more critical role. Companies offering health plans must consider location and primary care access for potential enrollees. While in past years a physician could establish an office in a location convenient for the doctor, today the consumer increasingly dictates the role of place in the marketing mix.

While the obvious factors of location and layout are considered, hours, access, obstacles, waits for appointments, claims payment, etc., should also be included in the notion of place. In most cases, the negative "place" aspects of the encounter impose costs such as lost time, frustration in finding the service site, parking fees, boredom, or other emotional burdens. Positive "place" aspects usually merely avoid such costs, as when a physician who offers early morning or evening hours enables patients to obtain care on the way to or from work, and thus avoid time off from work, travel costs, and lost wages.

Promotion

"Promotion" is the fourth "P" of the marketing mix. Promotion refers to any means of informing the marketplace that the organization has developed a response to meet its needs. Promotion involves a range of tactics involving publicity, advertising, and personal selling. The promotional mix refers to the various communication techniques such as advertising, personal selling, sales promotion, and public relations/product publicity available to the marketer to achieve specific goals. The promotional mix refers to the combination of the various marketing techniques utilized by a marketer.

The application of the traditional four Ps of the marketing mix to healthcare is considered problematic by many observers. Some consider these dimensions of marketing inappropriate for a service-oriented industry like healthcare. The uncomfortable fit between the four Ps of marketing and healthcare has even led some to pronounce the "death" of the four Ps and suggest their replacement with some other, more appropriate model in healthcare. (Box 2.1 discusses the importance of relationship development in healthcare.)

Box 2.1 Marketing as relationship development

There was a time in healthcare when the bulk of marketing was geared toward "making the sale," getting that customer in the door, or signing them up for an affinity program. Too much attention was paid to getting a $500 sale rather than obtaining a customer-for-life who would ultimately spend $250,000 on healthcare. The *real* goal of marketing should be to establish a relationship that will pay long-term dividends.

A useful example of marketing-as-relationship-development is the patient satisfaction survey conducted after discharge. Ostensibly, the intent of the survey is to measure customer satisfaction in order to improve service in the future. But the simple process of collecting satisfaction data can be viewed as an opportunity for developing a relationship with that patient and his or her family. Seeking input from customers and otherwise engaging them in dialogue can serve multiple purposes. Seen in this light, the $15 that seemed high for a completed satisfaction questionnaire doesn't look like much of an investment for solidifying a relationship with a potential lifelong customer.

Promotion in healthcare is different because we are not just trying to make a sale, but we are trying to get the consumer to go to the right place at the right time to receive the right care. From the outset, promotional efforts should educate, instruct, and direct consumers to the proper place for their care. In healthcare relationships with consumers are based on the notion that each individual customer is getting exactly what they need the first time and in the most efficient manner possible. Consumers must believe that we will live up to our end of the bargain in providing the most appropriate care. It is this educational element that sets healthcare apart from marketing in other industries.

Relationship marketing, of necessity, pays careful attention to customer needs and service delivery and is characterized by: (1) a focus on customer retention, (2) an orientation towards product benefits rather than product features, (3) a long-term view of the relationship, (4) maximum emphasis on customer commitment and contact, (5) development of on-going relationships, (6) multiple employee/customer contacts, (7) an emphasis on key account relationship management, and (8) an emphasis on trust.

Chapter 3
The Marketing Process

Marketing – regardless of the form it takes – is not a discrete activity but a process. The end result of this process – a print or electronic ad, a telemarketing campaign, or a celebrity endorsement – represents a fraction of the total effort involved in designing, developing and implementing the marketing activity. This chapter outlines the process involved in creating an effective marketing initiative.

Steps in the Process

Applying the term "process" to healthcare marketing implies that there are certain procedures to be followed and sequential steps to be completed. Although every marketing campaign may not follow the exact same steps, there are certain parts of the process that must be completed and these are discussed below.

Framing the Situation

Any marketer is going to want to know certain things before even considering the development of a marketing initiative. He or she is going to want to know something about the organization. Is it new or old, large or small, sleet of foot or molasses slow along with many other characteristics? A marketer is going to ask about the good or service that is being promoted. In basic terms: What are we selling? As noted in the previous chapter, what is being sold could be a product or service, an organization or an idea.

Regardless of the nature of the product being offered, the marketer is going to want to know something about existing marketing efforts. Does the product already have a presence in the market? Are there previous or current marketing initiatives underway? How effective (or ineffective) have previous marketing efforts been? The last thing the marketer wants to do is muddy the waters, so an understanding of the existing marketing situation is critical. (See Box 3.1 for questions to ask about existing marketing activities.)

Box 3.1 Assessing existing marketing activities

Few marketing initiatives are going to represent truly "virgin" territory. So, when a new marketing campaign is suggested, any marketer is going to want to know what marketing efforts have previously been undertaken vis-à-vis the product to be marketed. The questions below represent a starting point in terms of determining the status of existing marketing activities:

- How well has the product (service, organization, idea) been defined?
- To what extent do members of the organization see this as a distinct product (service, organization, idea)?
- How much thought has been given to the packaging of this product (service, organization, idea)?
- What promotional materials have been developed to support this product (service, organization, idea)?
- What promotional activities have been previously implemented for this product (service, organization, idea)?
- Who if anyone has been given responsibility for the marketing of this product (service, organization, idea)?
- Can the impact of previous marketing activities be measured (and, if so, what can be determined)?

The marketer will also want to determine something about the environment in which the marketing activity will take place. The shape of the healthcare landscape should be determined and the organization's place in it specified as completely as possible. Is the environment supportive of the organization and its programs? Is the healthcare market growing or shrinking? Is the market well insured or otherwise able to pay for services?

The marketer needs to determine who competes with the organization doing the marketing, as well as what other products out there vie for the consumer's attention. What alternatives exist to the product in the marketplace? What products are competing with this one, and how have they positioned themselves in the market?

Stating Assumptions

"Assumptions" are the understandings that drive the planning process, and, if they are not specified early in the process, the marketing team may find itself well down the road holding conflicting notions of what the project is really about. Assumptions can relate to demographic trends, reimbursement practices, the competitive situation and any number of other aspects of the healthcare system. Assumptions should be made about the audience that is being targeted, the nature of the population, the political climate, other options for services, and so forth.

Some assumptions can – and should – be stated at the outset of the planning process. Others will be developed as information is collected and more in-depth knowledge gained concerning the community, its healthcare needs, and its resources. These assumptions, regardless when stated, should inform the rest of the process.

Reviewing Available Data

In framing the situation related to the marketing initiative, the marketer will have asked some basic questions and received responses from managers and others familiar with the organization and its products. That information represents a good start, but any marketer will want to get "harder" data before moving forward with a marketing initiative.

There are a variety of sources from which such data can be obtained and these sources are discussed in detail in the chapter on marketing research. Both published and unpublished reports may be available from internal and external sources. A number of federal health information clearinghouses and websites also provide information, products, materials, and sources of further assistance for specific health subjects.

A helpful first step in assessing the problem may be to access the appropriate websites and the health department to obtain information on the health issue being addressed. There are standard sources of data that most marketers will know about: census data for demographics, health department data for fertility and mortality statistics, state agencies for facilities information and utilization data, and so forth. These secondary sources of data typically go a long way toward fleshing out the context in which the marketing will take place.

Gaps in available information should be noted and sources of additional data identified. The marketer may find that the data gathered do not give enough insight into the market situation thus calling for additional research, or that other important information about the target audiences may be unavailable or outdated. The marketer should take advantage of any readily available data on the organizations, its products and services, the healthcare environment and the competitive situation, and fill in the data gaps as necessary.

Profiling the Intended Audience(s)

The identification of the intended audiences starts with a review of the epidemiology of the problem. This effort will determine the extent of the marketing challenge to be addressed, the segments of the population that are most affected, the characteristics of those at greatest risk, and any other factors that might facilitate a resolution to the marketing problem.

Target audiences can be carved out of broad population groups and defined more narrowly based on characteristics such as attitudes, demographics, geographic region, or patterns of behavior. Examples might include physically inactive adolescents, heavy smokers with low education and income levels, or urban African-American men with hypertension. The target audience's ability and willingness to respond in the desired manner affects the role of marketing as the initiative moves forward.

Setting Marketing Goals

The marketing goal represents the generalized accomplishment that the organization would like to achieve through the planned initiative. The goal or goals that are established for the marketing plan should reflect the information generated by means of the background research and be in keeping with the organization's mission statement and strategic plan.

The goal of the marketing initiative should be broad in scope and limited in detail. It should be stated in a form such as: To establish Hospital X as the top-of-mind facility in this market area. Or, for a service-specific initiative, it might read: To dominate the niche for occupational medicine in this market area.

Formulating the Marketing Strategy

Somewhere during this process, a decision must be made with regard to the choice of strategy. The strategy refers to the generalized approach to marketing that is best suited for achieving the stated goal. The strategy should provide overall direction for the initiative, fit the available resources, minimize any potential resistance, resonate with the appropriate target audience, and, ultimately, frame the process for accomplishing the goals of the marketing initiative.

While the precise strategic approach may not be specified at this point, the options can be narrowed. This will serve to focus subsequent planning activities by eliminating strategies that are not considered appropriate. For example, it may have been determined that the target population must be educated on the issues prior to attempting behavioral change. In that case, the strategy would focus – initially at least – on education and information dissemination rather than "sales."

Once a marketing strategy has been established, all program elements should be compatible with it. This means every project task should contribute to reaching the established objectives and be designed to reach the intended audiences; all messages and materials should incorporate the benefits and other information from the strategy statement.

Defining Marketing Objectives

Objectives refer to the specific targets to be reached in support of goal attainment. While goals are general statements, objectives should be very specific and stated in clear and concise terms. Any concepts referenced in an objective must be operationalizable and measurable. Objectives must also be time bound, with clear deadlines established for their accomplishment. Finally, they must be amenable to evaluation.

Several objectives may be specified related to the goal of the marketing initiative. Four or five would not be uncommon, although many more than that becomes unwieldy (especially if more than one goal is being considered). Some decision may have to be made with regard to the number and priority of the objectives. The potential barriers and the likely consequences – intended and unintended – should be considered.

It is important to create achievable objectives, and many marketing efforts "fail" because the original objectives were unreasonable. It is virtually impossible, for example, to increase a hospital's market share in a major market by more than a couple of percentage points, and any higher goal should be considered unrealistic. If a numerical goal for a particular objective is to be specified, the marketer should determine how much change a marketing initiative can reasonably be expected to effect. Without measurable objectives, there is no way to demonstrate that a program has succeeded or is making progress along the way. (See Box 5.5 in Chapter 5 for examples of goals and objectives.)

Developing the Promotional Mix

There are a variety of ways in which a product might be promoted, and the ways that are selected for a particular situation constitute the promotional mix. The promotional technique selected should reflect the strategy that has been adopted, the nature of the organization, the type of product, and relevant characteristics of the community. Importantly, the likely effectiveness of any given technique should be considered in view of these factors.

Promotional appeals might be aimed at the emotions, intellect, or pocketbooks of the target audience. The best approach depends on the intended audience's preferences, the type of information being communicated and, ultimately, what the initiative hopes to accomplish. In any case, the type of appeal employed should reflect the strategy that has been chosen. The research conducted earlier should provide insights into the appropriate type of appeal and its format, timing and channels for distribution. (Box 3.2 discusses the testing of promotional materials.)

Materials Developing

Developing and pretesting messages and materials are important because they indicate early in the process which messages will be most effective with the intended audiences. Knowing this will save your organization time and money. Positive results from pretesting can also generate early buy-in from others in the organization.

Although message and materials development and production are often time-consuming and costly, these represent a critical step in the development of a marketing

---

Box 3.2 Testing marketing concepts

The more effort that goes into the testing of marketing concepts on the front end, the less likely there will be disappointing results on the back end. Some rules to consider in testing marketing concepts include:

- Become as smart as possible about the target audience before developing materials.
- Consider other efforts that have been made to promote similar products to similar audiences.
- Involve a variety of perspectives in materials development (including those of the target audience).
- Provide a variety of options for use during the pretesting.
- Don't attempt to influence responses during concept testing.
- Test concepts under conditions that resemble those under which the audience exposure will actually take place.

---

initiative. Given the magnitude of this task, existing marketing materials (booklets, leaflets, posters, public service announcements, videotapes) should be inventoried. If not directly applicable, they may serve as a foundation for subsequent materials development.

Once effective message concepts have been identified, it is possible to determine the formats (e.g., brochure, videotape) that will best suit the initiative. These materials should be evaluated in terms of:

- The nature of the message (e.g., its complexity, sensitivity, style)
- The function of the message (e.g., to call attention to an issue or to teach a new skill)
- The activities and channels previously selected
- The budget and other available resources

The development of new materials typically represents a major expenditure. Formats should be chosen that your program can afford and care taken to not spend disproportionately on materials development. Knowledge of the intended audience should be used to combine, adapt, and devise new ways to get the message across. Input should be sought from the intended audience or partners with regard to decisions about materials.

Determining the Channels

The channels available for the delivery of a promotional message continue to grow in number and complexity. The relative attraction of various channels for the consuming public is constantly changing. It might help to start with some broad categories of distribution channels and narrow options down as more information about the target audience is obtained.

Interpersonal channels (e.g., physicians, friends, family members, counselors, parents), may be able to present health messages in a familiar context. These channels are more likely to be trusted and influential than media sources. Developing messages, materials, and links for interpersonal channels may require time; but these channels are often effective for affecting attitudes, skills, and behavior/behavioral intent. Influence through interpersonal contacts may work best when the individual is already familiar with the message, for example, from hearing it through mass media exposure.

Group channels (e.g., brown bag lunches at work, classroom activities, church group discussions, neighborhood gatherings, and club meetings) may be the best way to reach some intended audiences. Health messages can be designed for groups with specific things in common, such as workplace, school, church, club affiliations, or favorite activities, and these channels add the benefits of group discussion and affirmation of the messages.

Impersonal channels such as the electronic and print media (including the Internet) typically consume the bulk of the effort (and money) invested in marketing. While all forms of mass media have some potential for healthcare marketing, the pros and cons of each must be carefully considered. Network television may not be very useful for promoting a local organization but selected cable channels may be, while radio may be an effective means of disseminating certain messages. Newspapers may reach that demographic segment that has not gone over to cyberspace, while high-end magazines may reach the target audience for elective procedures.

Extensive research has been conducted (in other industries) on the sources of information, communication patterns, and media preferences for virtually any target audience. This information should be consulted when decisions are being made with regard to distribution channels.

Implementing the Marketing Campaign

The marketing process creates a road map which the marketing staff uses to move the initiative to where it needs to be. The transition from planning to implementation involves a hand-off from the planning team to the management team. Implementation must occur at several different levels and within different divisions of the organization. For this reason, the implementation of the campaign requires a high level of coordination.

In order to approach implementation systematically, the marketing team should develop a detailed project plan and an implementation matrix to support it. An implementation matrix can be developed using a spreadsheet and should lay out who is to do what and when they are to do it. The matrix should list every action called for by the plan, breaking each action down into tasks, if appropriate. For each action or task the responsible party should be identified, along with any secondary parties that should be involved in this activity. The matrix should indicate resource requirements (in terms of

Table 3.1 Sample implementation matrix

Marketing Plan Implementation		
Task/Subtask	Start date	End date
Market research		
Market profile	3/1/2005	4/15/2005
Demand estimates	3/15/2005	4/15/2005
Employer analysis	3/15/2005	4/15/2005
Employer targeting	5/1/2005	On-going
Partner needs assessment	4/15/2005	5/1/505
Marketing evaluation	4/1/2005	On-going
Brand development		
Brand conceptualization	4/15/2005	5/15/2005
Brand copy	6/1/2005	6/15/2005
Product branding opportunities	5/15/2005	6/15/2005
Branding partner identification	6/1/2005	7/1/2005
Brand materials preparation	6/15/2005	7/15/2005
Corporate (collateral) materials		
Copy preparation	4/1/2005	4/15/2005
Finalize brochure	5/1/2005	5/1/2005
Print brochure	5/15/2005	6/1/2005
Letterhead	6/1/2005	6/15/2005
Business cards	6/1/2005	6/15/2005
Web site content	5/1/2005	6/15/2005
Posters	5/15/2005	6/15/2005
Media kit	6/1/2005	6/15/2005
Public relations		
Copy preparation	4/1/2005	5/1/2005
Media list	4/15/2005	5/1/2005
Media contact strategy	5/1/2005	5/15/2005
Event list	4/15/2005	5/1/2005

staff time, money and other requirements). The start and end dates for this activity should be identified. Any prerequisites for accomplishing this task should be identified at the outset and factored into the project plan. Finally, benchmarks should be established that allow the planning team to determine when the activity has been completed. (Table 3.1 provides on example of a simple implementation matrix.)

Launching the Campaign

Before the launch of a marketing campaign, it is important to plan for distribution, promotion, and evaluation. This requires the marketing staff to develop a launch plan, produce sufficient quantities of materials, and prepare for the tasks that support the launch. The nature of the initiative might dictate a quiet, low-key launch or call for a major kick-off event. Kickoff events are an excellent way to develop relationships with people who may be willing to get involved in the program.

In order to enhance media coverage for a kickoff event, a number of steps can be taken. The organization might create a news "hook" or angle that makes the event newsworthy, informing the media of your event in a timely manner, creating media kits to facilitate accurate reporting of the issue and including the full range of appropriate media. Some media may have a greater incentive to use a feature story or news item than general newspapers or regular TV stations, and they can ensure an audience at a press conference if the mainstream media don't show up. Public relations professionals typically know which media meet which of these needs.

Managing the Campaign

The primary tasks involved in managing a marketing campaign include monitoring activities, staff, and budget; problem solving; process evaluation; measuring audience response; and revising plans and operations. The implementation plan developed to manage the campaign should indicate how and when resources will be needed, when specific events will occur, and at what points efforts will be assessed.

It is often possible to correct problems quickly if they can be identified. For example, if the public is being asked to call you for more information, a simple form (electronic or manual) for telephone operators to use to record the questions asked and the answers given would be useful if not essential. Every marketing initiative should be monitored to review responses to identify inquiry patterns, assure that correct or adequate information is being given, and determine whether more or different information may be needed. Of course, managing the budget is a critical requirement for any marketing initiative. (Box 3.3 provides a checklist useful for monetoring the campaign.)

Evaluating the Campaign

Evaluation is necessary to determine the efficiency of the process and the effectiveness of the initiative. Process evaluation measures efficiency by evaluating systems, procedures, communication processes, and other factors that contribute to the efficient operation of a program. Outcome evaluation focuses more on end results and measures the effectiveness of the initiative in achieving its objectives. The notion of evaluating the marketing project should be top of mind on the first day of the process, and the means for evaluation should be built into the process itself.

Data collection should be carefully planned on the frontend in order to measure progress toward project objectives. Benchmarkes should be established and constantly monitored. (More information of evaluating marketing efforts is provided in Chapter 12.)

Box 3.3 Marketing process checklist

The following checklist might be useful to the marketer in determining whether the marketing process has been properly carried out:

- ☑ Define the marketing problem
- ☑ Define the product
- ☑ Determine the status of the product in the market
- ☑ Identify and profile the target market
- ☑ State assumptions
- ☑ Set marketing goal(s)
- ☑ Formulate a strategy
- ☑ Specify and refine objectives
- ☑ Determine the promotional mix
- ☑ Develop and test promotional materials
- ☑ Launch the campaign
- ☑ Implement the campaign
- ☑ Evaluate the campaign

Chapter 4
Marketing Research

Marketing research addresses the nature of the product or service, the characteristics of consumers, the size of the potential market, the nature of competitors, and any number of other essential pieces of the marketing puzzle. This chapter describes the various aspects of marketing research and familiarizes the reader with the basic skills required to carry out this activity.

The Importance of Research

"Marketing research," often used interchangeably with "market research," is usually thought to encompass market research, product research, pricing research, promotional research, and distribution research. Marketing research is an important component of the marketing process and should represent the starting point for any marketing initiative. Beyond the obvious reason for conducting marketing research – the gathering of critical information – there are other good reasons to invest in this activity. Perhaps the most important is the contribution that research makes to the decision-making process. Decision making in healthcare increasingly relies upon accurate, timely, and detailed data to supplement the knowledge base acquired through experience. In this way, the marketer and administration can combine their resources to generate market intelligence.

The type and amount of research undertaken during the marketing process is dictated by a number of factors, including the kind of marketing initiative being formulated, the nature of the organization, the available resources, and the intended use of the findings. A critical skill for the marketer is the ability to determine the type and scope of research appropriate for a particular marketing initiative.

When to Do Marketing Research

Marketing research is often triggered by some event or situation. A need is identified and research is initiated. In an ideal world, however, the research necessary to support marketing would be an ongoing function within the organization. It is not practical to initiate discrete research projects from scratch to support every marketing initiative. In other words, effective marketing research is proactive rather than reactive. By the time most organizations can mount a data collection initiative the marketing campaign period is likely to be over. With research capabilities already in place, it is possible to routinely analyze market, trends such as changes in physician referral, shifts in admissions, by specialty or emerging market niches. Conducting research after the "horse has escaped from the barn" is not likely to be very useful.

Data Dimensions in Marketing Research

The data collected during marketing research can be categorized along a number of different dimensions. By categorizing data in this manner, some organization is introduced into the data management process. Some of the most important dimensions are addressed in the sections below.

Community Versus Organizational Data

The compilation of health data can be approached at two different levels, the community level and the organizational level. The former involves the analysis of community-wide health data, whether the "community" is the nation, a state, a county or a planning district. The latter focuses on data specific to a particular organization. Community-level data focus on top-of-the-organization statistics as opposed to detailed internal data for organizations. The emphasis is likely to be on overall patterns of health service delivery and on dominant practice patterns than on the details of the operation of specific organizations. Thus, community-level research will generate data on such phenomena as patient flow into and out of the service area, levels of overcapacity or under-capacity affecting the area's health facilities, and the adequacy of various types of biomedical equipment within the service area.

At the organization level, data analysis focuses on the characteristics and concerns of specific corporate entities such as hospitals, physician groups, and health plans. These data provide details on the organization's operation vis-à-vis the activities of competitors and other healthcare organizations within the market area. They would include details on competing specialty practices (e.g., patient volume, market share, procedures performed) rather than more general data on the health service area. It is likely that both community- and organization-level data will be utilized for most marketing research, and the nature of the marketing initiative will dictate the relative importance of the two types of data.

Internal Versus External Data

Healthcare organizations routinely generate a large volume of data as a by-product of their normal operations. These include data related to patient characteristics, utilization patterns, referral streams, financial transactions, personnel and other types of information. To the extent that these data can be extracted from internal data management systems, they serve as a rich source of information on the organization and its operations. Internal data are usually compiled through an *internal audit*.

Data on the internal characteristics of the organization typically include information on patient characteristics, utilization trends, staffing levels, and financial trends, among others. The internal audit typically includes analysis of the organization's structure, processes, customers and resources. The internal audit may compile data produced by the organization's data management systems (e.g., patient activity reports), although some situations may require custom data compilation.

Most of the data collection effort on the part of marketers will be directed toward external data. As healthcare providers have become market driven and the emphasis has shifted to marketing planning, the interest in external data of all types has grown. These data provide market intelligence on issues external to the organization and include information on national, state and local trends in healthcare delivery, financing and regulation. Marketers need to be aware of developments in the local market that will affect their initiatives. They particularly need to have an understanding of the characteristics of other healthcare organizations within the market area, especially competitors.

Primary Versus Secondary Data

Primary data collection involves the use of surveys, focus groups, observational methods and other techniques for the stated purpose of obtaining information on a specific topic. Secondary data refers to data gathered for some other purpose besides planning, marketing, or business development but that is nevertheless of value in the formulation of marketing strategy.

Secondary data is the bread-and-butter of marketing research and should be used whenever possible. Indeed, the most effective marketing researchers are those who know how to find, access and interpret secondary data. Many of the sources of data used by marketers in other industries can be accessed by healthcare marketers, although it may sometimes be necessary to seek out health-specific data sources.

Primary research is likely to be used when certain types of data cannot be acquired from secondary sources. For example, in collecting data to support marketing for a new health service, an analyst may: (1) examine hospital records for information relating to past introductions of similar services (secondary data); (2) conduct a set of interviews to determine current consumer attitudes about the service (primary survey data); and (3) conduct a pilot study in which consumer perception of the proposed service is measured (primary experimental data).

If primary research is deemed necessary, the researcher should determine whether qualitative or quantitative research (or both) is required. Qualitative research is more subjective in nature and employed when an in-depth understanding of an issue that involves attitudes and perceptions is required. Qualitative methods include observation, interviews and focus groups. Quantitative methods are employed when it is necessary to obtain "hard data" from a large number of subjects for purposes of detailed analysis. Quantitative methods emphasize survey research and may involve experimental or quasi-experimental methods.

Geographic Level

Healthcare marketers are likely to operate at different levels of geography depending on the characteristics of the marketing initiative. The type of organization and the nature of the service area will determine the level of geography at which data are required. A large specialty group is likely to draw patients from a wide geographic area covering several counties; in this case, the county is probably the best unit for data collection. A family practitioner in a solo practice is likely to serve a fairly circumscribed service area that exists within a particular county. In this case, the ZIP code may be the level at which data would be collected and analyzed.

The choice of geographic unit for the analysis is important not only because of its implications for the service area under study, but because different types of data are available for different geographies. For many types of information, the county may offer the most extensive range of data and, generally, the smaller the unit of geography the less data is available. While use of the ZIP code or census tract as the unit of geography may allow for more precise delineation of the service area, access to certain types of data may be limited. Thus, there is likely to be a tradeoff related to the specification of the service area and the types of data that are available. (Box 4.1 describes the varires geographic units utilized in marketing research.)

Temporal Dimension

One other dimension of data that needs to be taken into consideration is the temporal dimension. Health professionals typically think in terms of current data – that is, data that relate to the present timeframe or, at least, to the immediate past (e.g., the last set of lab tests). From a marketing perspective, however, current data are important but, in some ways, are less useful than future data and even historical data. The value of current data rests with its ability to provide a baseline against which past and future figures can be compared. "Future" data refers to data that describe conditions at some point in the future.

Box 4.1 Geographic units for market analysis

Marketing researchers should be familiar with the various types of geographic units utilized in collecting market data. The highest level of geography that might be utilized for market analysis (assuming the organization involved is not a multinational corporation) would be the entire *nation*. While few organizations today actually view the national population as a realistic market, statistics on the characteristics of the United States population are often utilized for comparative purposes.

The next lowest level would be the regional level of the United States. The Bureau of the Census divides the nation into four grand *regions* (Northeast, Southeast, Midwest and West) based on groupings of the 50 states. The Census Bureau further subdivides the four regions into divisions of a few states each. These divisions are often useful if data are required at the sub-region level. These regions generally do not coincide with any meaningful healthcare service areas, but are useful for general market research purposes.

The *state* level is effectively the largest geographic unit utilized by most market researchers in healthcare, since it is the largest unit of geography that is manageable for market analysis purposes. Many organizations (e.g., health maintenance organizations) are chartered to operate in specific states and a substantial amount of data is generated at the state level.

The next lowest level of geography, and the most frequently utilized "building block" for delineating market areas, is the *county* (or county equivalent in some states). A wide variety of data is available at the county level, since state and federal agencies typically report most of their statistics at this level. County agencies themselves also generate a great deal of data.

In cases where the organization's service area is smaller than a county and others where portions of more than one county may comprise the service area, the *ZIP code* may be used. Zip codes are based on the postal distribution areas of the U.S. Postal Service and, as such, are familiar to most business decision makers. Unlike the geographic units previously discussed, ZIP codes do not constitute formal government boundaries.

While zip code-level data is adequate for most market analysis purposes, there may be cases when an even lower level of geography is required. *Census tracts* have been established by the Bureau of the Census for data collection purposes and ideally contain between 2,000 and 4,000 residents. The census tract is the unit for which the most extensive and detailed data are collected during national censuses.

In the rare cases in which a lower level of geography is desired, the use of census *block groups* or even census *blocks* may be desirable. A census block is simply a square block of residential land, typically delineated by streets on four sides. Block groups represent an aggregation of census blocks.

(continued)

Box 4.1 (continued)

The use of various units of geography has been facilitated by the availability of desktop mapping packages and the more sophisticated geographic information systems. An important feature of these software applications is the ability to "geocode" addresses to specific latitudes and longitudes. Once an address (e.g., for a patient or a facility) has been geocoded, the county, ZIP code, or census tract for that site can be easily determined. This feature greatly facilitates any spatial analysis performed using the above units of geography.

Box 4.2 Marketing research questions

The marketer or project director will typically answer the following questions when developing the research project:

- How much of the information required is available from secondary data sources?
- Are there data gaps that call for primary research and, if so, what type of research is appropriate?
- If primary research is required, should qualitative or quantitative methods be utilized?
- To what extent will it be necessary to collect data on the organization doing the marketing (internal) versus data on the environment (external)?
- What is the appropriate geographic level at which the relevant data should be compiled?
- Do we have the ability to collect the required data or should outside resources be utilized?

Market researchers may collect historical data on the community or the organization in order to extrapolate past trends into the future. Thus, historical patterns of population growth, hospital admissions, and disease prevalence can provide the basis for predicting future trends. Since actual future data do not exist, efforts must be made to generate projections of future conditions relevant to the community or the healthcare organization. To that end, increasing emphasis is being placed on the production of "synthetic" estimates of future populations, service demands and utilization patterns. The growing interest in predictive modeling among health plans and other care managers is encouraging the development of techniques for predicting future trends. (Box 4.2 presents questions to be ask while organizing the research effort.)

Dimensions of Marketing Research

Foundational Research

Marketing research can take a variety of forms, and it is not always a formal, expensive process. Any type of information gathering on the marketplace constitutes marketing research. Although the focus is on the formal aspects of market research, more casual approaches such as observation and mystery shoppers have a role in healthcare marketing research.

In marketing research the first step typically involves developing a generalized understanding of the community or organization for which marketing is occurring. For any marketing initiative, information on the product or service is required, as well as information on the market area and its population.

A review of the existing literature is an obvious place to start the research process. "Literature" is used here in a very broad sense. In traditional research this typically refers to the professional journals in which the field's conventional wisdom is codified. The literature for health services marketing will include not only standard journals but newsletters, government reports, technical papers, professional meeting presentations, annual reports, and the publications of professional associations.

Today, marketers can gain access to the Internet for literature reviews and other sources of relevant information. Most bibliographic databases can be accessed through the Internet and any number of other sources – some of them quite serendipitous – can be uncovered by accessing the World Wide Web. Another type of electronic "literature review" involves the growing volume of e-mail exchanges among the informal network of health professionals. An increasing amount of health-related data is becoming available via the World Wide Web and the Internet is becoming a standard research tool.

The data collection process can take a variety of forms, but will typically involve both primary data collection and the use of secondary data. Secondary data are virtually always collected first because they are likely to be readily available without much in the way of additional expense.

Sources of Data

Secondary data refers to data that have been previously collected for some purpose that may or may not relate to the project at hand. In fact, much of the data utilized in marketing research was compiled for administrative, clinical or financial uses without any notion that the information would be utilized for marketing purposes. Secondary data collected within the organization is usually acquired through an internal audit. Secondary data collected on factors external to the organization is usually acquired through an external audit or environmental assessment.

Internal Audit

In performing the internal audit a number of different aspects of the organization should be examined. Some or all of the following aspects of the organization would be of interest at this point:

Services/products. What are the services that are provided and/or the products that are produced? What are the characteristics of these services and products?

Customer characteristics. How many customers does the organization have and what are their characteristics? What are the demographic characteristics that are most pertinent? Where do patients reside and what is the "reach" of the organization? What is the case mix and payor mix of current customers?

Utilization patterns. What is the volume of services and products consumed by the organization's customers? How does this volume breakdown by product line or procedure?

Pricing structure. How is pricing determined for the organization's services and products? How does this price structure compare with that of competitors or the industry average? How price sensitive are the goods and services offered?

Locations. To what extent are operations centralized or decentralized? How many satellite locations are operated and how were their locations chosen? Are there markets that are not being served by existing outlets?

Referral relationships. How are customers referred to the organization? To what extent are formal referral relationships in place?

Existing marketing activities. What, if any, marketing activities are already in play for the product being promoted? To what extent have these efforts been effective? How well has the product been received by the target audience? (Box 4.3 provides a checklist for the internal audit.)

External Audit

The external audit or environmental assessment involves the collection and analysis of data external to the organization. The assessment can take place at the national level, the regional level (if appropriate), the state level, and ultimately at the level of the community under study.

Broad societal trends should be analyzed and their implications for the local environment considered. These societal trends should include demographic trends, economic considerations, lifestyle trends, and even shifts in attitudes. National trends in lifestyles (e.g., fitness) and health-related fads (e.g., cosmetic surgery) should be considered. Trends in consumer attitudes are another area of inquiry.

Developments in the healthcare industry should be examined to identify any trends at the national or state levels that are likely to affect the local community. These could include trends in financial arrangements, changing organizational

Box 4.3 Checklist for the internal audit

The internal audit can provide a great deal of information concerning the organization and even offer insights into the external environment. While the project – and the availability of useful data – will determine the content of the internal audit, the following list provides examples of the types of data that might be extracted up from the data systems of a healthcare organization.

Services/products
    Clinical services provided
    Nonclinical services provided
    Products sold
    Locations/distribution outlets

Customer characteristics
    Demographic characteristics
    Diagnoses
    Financial category/payor mix
    Patient origin
    Psychographic characteristics
    Socioeconomic characteristics

Utilization trends
    Patient visits
    Patient encounters
    Hospital admissions
    Diagnostic tests performed
    Treatments provided
    Referral patterns
    Patient satisfaction

Financial data
    Pricing
    Charges billed
    Revenue collected
    Cost of services
    Profit margin/net revenue

Staffing
    Number of employees
    Breakdown by category
    Personnel expenses
    Other expenses
    Marketing expenses

Box 4.4 External audit checklist

This checklist presents the categories of data that could conceivably be collected as part of the external audit. The intensity with which this checklist is used will depend on the nature of the organization and the type of marketing initiative envisioned.

Societal (national) trends
  Demographic trends
  Economic trends
  Lifestyle trends
Health industry trends
  Organizational developments
  Financial/reimbursement trends
  Technology developments
  Diagnosis/treatment trends
Regulatory trends
  Political trends
  Regulatory developments
  Legal developments
Market characteristics
  Community type
  Geographic position
  Demographic trends
      Age
      Sex
      Race
      Ethnicity
      Marital status
      Family structure
      Educational level
      Socioeconomic characteristics
      Income level
      Labor force characteristics
      Industry profile
      Occupational characteristics
      Insurance coverage
      Psychographic/lifestyle characteristics
Health status
  Fertility trends
  Morbidity trends
  Mortality trends

(continued)

Box 4.4 (continued)

Health behavior
   Informal health behavior
   Formal health behavior
      Hospital statistics
      Physician visits
      Emergency room visits
      Drug utilization
      Other utilization indicators

Market area resources
   Facilities
   Programs/services
   Personnel
   Equipment
   Networks/relationships
   Sources of funding

structures within the delivery system, or the introduction of new treatment modalities. Organizational developments such as the emergence of large national for-profit chains and the establishment of business coalitions should be considered. Regulatory, political and legal developments at the national and state level should be examined.

Developments in the area of technology can exert a major influence on the course of the healthcare system. The introduction of new drugs has changed the manner in which behavioral health problems are addressed, refinements in biomedical equipment have made home care more feasible for a range of conditions, and microsurgical techniques have contributed to the shift of care from the inpatient to the outpatient setting. Developments in information technology will continue to have a vital impact on healthcare.

Financing issues may be impacted by all levels of government as well as by private sector third-party payors. Trends in reimbursement characterizing government-sponsored health programs and managed care plans need to be considered. Any changes in reimbursement may have significant implications for healthcare providers. (Box 4.4 presents a checklist for the external audit).

Profiling the Market

The internal and external audits establish the backdrop against which further analysis takes place. The next step in the data collection process involves developing baseline data on the community. These baseline data provide the foundation for the planning process, the basis for any future comparisons, and the yardstick by which the success of the planning process will be measured. This process identifies the who, what, when, where and how of the community and its healthcare system.

The *community type* should also be a consideration when collecting baseline data. Whether the dominant community type within the planning area is urban, suburban or rural will have important implications for both health status and health behavior. Not only will the circumstances surrounding the health of the population be different for different community types, but the challenge of marketing within different community types exists.

In profiling the market area, *demographic data* serve as the foundation for most market analysis. Not only are demographic data important for profiling the community, but they serve as the basis for the calculation of a number of statistics relevant for marketing research. While an understanding of the demographic composition of the target population is important in its own right, this information is also essential for identifying the prevalence of health conditions and determining utilization patterns within the community.

Psychographic data should be collected that reflect the values, attitudes and lifestyles that characterize the target population. Psychographic factors are particularly important in examining attitudes towards one's health and the likelihood of involvement in healthy or unhealthy behaviors. Psychographic analysis can help determine the healthcare needs and priorities for a population subgroup. Similarly, the *attitudes* characterizing the population being marketed to along with is another dimension that must be considered the population's cultural preferences.

Data should be collected on a number of health indicators that reflect the health status of the population. This information would include *fertility* characteristics, *morbidity* data and *mortality* statistics. Morbidity data in particular indicate the type and level of health services demand.

Data on *health behavior* should be collected and this should include both informal and formal behaviors – formal activities such as physician visits, hospital admissions, and prescription drug consumption and informal actions related to diet, exercise, and risk-taking.

Once the healthcare needs and utilization patterns have been determined, the available *community resources* should be identified. Resources inventoried will range from facilities to programs and services to personnel to relationships. Facilities include hospitals, nursing homes and other institutions for the treatment of physical or mental illnesses. Programs and services refer to the types of care that are provided in these settings. Personnel should be identified in terms of type, number, characteristics and distribution and include physicians, nurses, mental health personnel and any other type of health professional relevant for the analysis. A thorough inventory of community health services should include a review of existing networks and relationships within the delivery system. An important aspect of the resource inventory relates the identification and profiling of any competitors to the organization.

An understanding of the manner in which health services are funded within the community should be considered. The payor mix discussed earlier is clearly a starting point for determining how the community pays for healthcare and, ultimately, the population's relative ability to pay for services. The extent to which health services reimbursement relies on government funding in the form of Medicare and Medicaid is important. The level of commitment of funds for public health and charity services is also an important consideration. Any unique sources of funding, such as state programs for categorical disease treatment, should be identified.

Primary Research

Virtually every marketing study is going to require the collection of primary data, since there are always going to be situations when the desired information is simply not available. The major advantage of primary data is that the information is collected for the particular problem or issue under investigation, making the data more directly relevant and current than most secondary data. Another major advantage is that primary data collection allows the organization to maintain the proprietary nature of the information collected and control the types of information elicited.

On the other hand, primary data collection can entail significant costs and require an extended period of time to complete. The administration of primary research may also require some fairly sophisticated skills that may not be available within the organization.

When initiating primary research activities, the means of data collection must be determined on the front end. The "right" data collection method depends on a number of factors. Several commonly used methods for collecting primary data are described below grouped into qualitative and quantitative categories.

Qualitative Techniques

Observation. Observational research involves techniques in which the actions and/or attributes of those being studied are observed either by another individual or through a mechanical recording device such as a video camera. Data collection by means of observation is performed according to specified rules based on stated objectives. Observational techniques are characterized as either participatory or nonparticipatory.

Observational methods are typically used in marketing research when data cannot be obtained through interviews or from secondary sources. This approach is particularly useful when a process is being analyzed. For example, a hospital might place a trained observer in its waiting area to observe the admitting process. Observers might track individual emergency patients from their initial encounter in the admitting area through their examination in the emergency room. Some organizations use a "mystery patient" approach as a means of collecting data through observational research.

Although observational data are useful in observing what people do, they cannot address *why* people behave in the way they do. Thus, it is often necessary to supplement observational research with personal interviews or some other form of data collection to determine the motivations underlying of the observed behavior.

Individual and Group Interviews. In-depth interviews typically involve one respondent and one interviewer. The in-depth interview is of value when the respondent must be probed regarding his or her answers. Complicated questions or questions that do not lend themselves to simple dichotomous responses often require personal interviews. The interview does not necessarily follow a defined set of questions that must be asked in a predetermined order, but probes as necessary to elicit the required information. In-depth interviews are sometimes referred to as "key informant" interviews. They typically last 30–45 min, but can last several hours.

Focus groups may be established for addressing a particular topic of interest under the direction of a professional moderator. The objective is to have people express their feelings or views related to a concept or a product. Opportunities for informal focus groups may arise admit in healthcare might include all persons working the same shift in a particular department or the families and friends of patients in the outpatient waiting room.

Focus groups can be used to provide insights that contribute to the formulation of issues and the development of subsequent research activities. As such, they are a useful supplement to the other types of research employed.

Quantitative Research

Most quantitative research involves some type of survey. Data collection for survey research has historically taken one of three common forms: mail-out surveys, personal interviews, and telephone interviews. Computerized interviews and fax-based surveys are also becoming common. Each of the forms of survey research that an organization might undertake is described below.

Mail Surveys. Mail surveys are a common method of administering sample surveys. Mail surveys involve the development of a survey instrument, the identification of an appropriate sample of respondents, and the mailing of survey forms to the sample. Returned survey forms are analyzed according to predetermined analytical techniques.

Mail surveys have the advantage of being a relatively inexpensive way to collect data. These surveys also provide anonymity to the respondent and eliminate potential interviewer bias. Mail is an efficient way to contact individuals who are dispersed over a large geographical area. For this reason, mail surveys are often used in healthcare to collect patient satisfaction data.

The disadvantages to this data collection method include low response rates, self administration, and lengthy turnaround times.

Face-to-Face Surveys. Personal (or face-to-face) surveys represent a valuable method for collecting data when the respondent must be probed regarding his or her answers. Complicated questions or questions that require explication on the part of the interviewer can best be handled in a face-to-face situation. These interviews are relatively short and involve a large number of respondents who are deemed to be representative of the population being studied. Personal interviews also require a lower level of interviewing skills and less substantive knowledge of the topic than in-depth interviews. The disadvantages of face-to-face surveys include their high cost, the potential for response bias, and the challenge of establishing a representative sample.

Telephone Interviews. Telephone interviews represent a quick way to acquire information. Using multiple interviewers in a telephone interview bank, considerable data can be acquired in a short timeframe. If the interviewers have some "hook," a high response rate can generally be obtained. Telephone interviewing allows for a reasonable degree of probing by the interviewer. However, it is reasonably easy for the respondent to terminate a telephone interview.

There is an inherent sampling bias with telephone interviews in that they require the respondent to have a telephone. While telephone ownership is high in this country, certain areas or populations may have significantly lower telephone ownership than the national average. Low-income populations and racial and ethnic minority groups, in particular, have lower than average levels of telephone installation.

The disadvantages of this method of data collection include the potential for sampling bias (due to lack of telephone service and/or the substitution of cell phones), potentially high refusal rates, and the inability of interviewers to pick up on visual cues that might be apparent in a face-to-face survey.

Computer-assisted telephone interviewing (CATI) has become increasingly common among survey researchers, and inexpensive software has made this technology available to most interviewers.

Computerized Interviews

Computer-based interviews have become increasingly popular as software has become more user friendly, and the general public has become more comfortable with computers. In computerized interviewing, the computer presents the survey items to the respondent on the screen in very much the same form it would take on a printed questionnaire.

On-site computerized interviewing is being utilized in more and more healthcare settings. The most frequent use to date is for collecting patient satisfaction data. After a clinic visit, for example, a respondent may be asked to sit down at a computer station and "fill out" the questionnaire that is shown on the screen. The more user-friendly systems allow the user to touch the appropriate response on the screen. Others may instruct the interviewee to strike certain keys on a keyboard.

This on-site approach to data collection has the advantage of capturing the information at a time when it is top of mind. It allows researchers to obtain responses from virtually every patient rather than relying on a sample. The provision of information is easy for the respondent, and the computer-assisted system often has the ability to modify itself during the course of the interview, edit the responses, and even perform analysis. Computerized interviewing saves time and resources and eliminates much of the paper involved in survey research. The results of the surveys can typically be obtained in hours if not minutes.

Table 4.1 Comparison of data collection methods for primary research

Method	Overall purpose	Advantages	Drawbacks
Observation	Collect information on behavior, activities and processes through structured observation	Able to observe phenomena in their natural setting while activities are taking place; allows direct observation rather than second-hand reports	Difficult to generate "hard" data for statistical analysis; difficult to interpret (especially the "why"); may required skilled observer
Interviews	Develop an understanding of (usually) a key respondent's attitudes or experiences and/or obtain in-depth information	Able to obtain detailed information on complicated issues and flesh out sketchy concepts; can probe for in-depth responses; basis for development of quantitative approaches	Difficult to generate "hard" data from interviews that reflect the perspectives of a small number of subjects; time consuming and difficult to interpret; may require a skilled, knowledgeable interviewer
Focus groups	Use structured discussion with a representative group of respondents to develop concepts, test ideas and flesh out issues	Ability to elicit various perspectives on an issue or idea; provides a more in-depth perspective than a survey; basis for the development of quantitative approaches	Difficult to generate "hard" data; hard to analyze responses; a skilled facilitator may be required; potential for "group think" or other dynamics that taint the responses
Surveys	Obtain a large amount of data from a large representative sample of a target population that can be subjected to statistical analysis	Ability to obtain a great deal of detail about a large number of people that can be generalized to a larger population	More complicated process than other forms of data collection; potential for poor questionnaire design and interviewer bias; increasingly expensive
Mail		Relatively inexpensive	Low response rate; relies on self-reporting
Telephone		Ability to probe	Gaining telephone access increasingly difficult; interviewer training issues
Face-to-face		Ability to probe and observe respondent behavior	Almost prohibitively expensive; interviewer training issues
Experiments	Use of a structured setting with a treatment group and control group to test hypotheses	Allows for the isolation of a phenomenon in a controlled setting that eliminates other influences; useful for testing concepts and materials	Difficult to establish a "pure" experiment especially in healthcare; limited ability to generalize results to a larger population

(continued)

Table 4.1 (continued)

Method	Overall purpose	Advantages	Drawbacks
Case studies	Develop an understanding of the operation of a program or the experiences of program participants through cross comparison of cases	Allows detailed description of a program's operation and/or the experiences of participants; identifies positive/negative attributes of the program; provides basis for development of quantitative methods	Time consuming to collect, organize and analyze material; limited ability to generalize to a larger population

The disadvantages of computer-based surveys include the need for a relatively short interview form, very simple and clearly worded survey items, and patients who are willing to cooperate, especially if they suffer from computer-phobia.

Some researchers have begun to administer surveys via the Internet, and the growing level of Internet penetration among the general public has made this medium increasingly popular. Assuming that the target population is "wired," data collection via the Internet is convenient and inexpensive. To date, this approach works best in the case of an existing network of customers, an advisory board, or other groupings that may already be linked by electronic mail, rather than for general consumers. As penetration rates increase and consumers become more familiar with this data collection approach, the use of the Internet for survey research will undoubtedly increase. (Table 4.1 presents comparative data on the various research methods.)

Sources of Data

Sources of Internal Data

Most health care organizations have immediate access to a "gold mine" of information – their own internal records. Health care organizations routinely generate a large amount of data as a by-product of their normal operations. Depending on the organization, data on patient characteristics, utilization trends, financial transactions, staffing, and a variety of other topics can be retrieved.

While data such as these are routinely collected by most healthcare organizations, they may not be as available or as useful as desired. Adequate computer technology must be in place in order to efficiently extract these data. These internal data may also have limitations due to the fact that they are seldom collected with marketing in mind. The fragmented nature of data processing within the hospital and the historical orientation toward function-specific databases have been major barriers to the adaptation of information systems to be responsive to a marketing orientation. As database marketing becomes more of a reality for hospitals and other health care providers, managing internal customer data (and the ability to interface them with external data) will become critical. To the extent that they are available and usable, internally generated data are essential for marketing researchers.

Data internal to a health care organization can be acquired in a number of ways. However, a systematic approach would involve the performance an *internal audit* that involves a review of the internal operations and organization of the health care organization as it relates to the marketing process. The internal audit examines the organization's *structure*, its *processes*, its *customers*, and its *resources*. The following types of internal data are typically accessed by marketing researchers:

- Patient Characteristics.
- Utilization Patterns.
- Financial Data.(including Insurance).
- Staffing and Other Resources.
- Referral Patterns.

The internal audit was discussed in more detail in Chapter 2.

Sources of External Data

There are numerous sources of data for marketing research available today and the number of sources continues to grow. The sections below group these sources into four main categories: government agencies, professional associations, private organizations, and commercial data vendors. It should be noted that the "products" available from these sources fall into different categories whose use depends on the needs of the researcher.

Government Agencies. Governments at all levels are involved in the generation, compilation, manipulation and/or dissemination of health-related data. The federal government, through the decennial census and related activities, is the world's largest processor of demographic data. Other federal agencies are major managers of data for the related topics of fertility, morbidity and mortality.

Through the National Center for Health Statistics, the Centers for Disease Control and Prevention, the National Institutes for Health, and other organizations, a large share of the nation's health data is generated. The Bureau of Health Resources (Department of Health and Human Services) maintains a master file of much of the health data compiled by the federal government entitled the *Area Resource File* (ARF).

Other federal sources outside of health-related agencies, such as the Bureau of Labor Statistics (e.g., health occupations) and the Department of Agriculture (e.g., nutritional data), create databases of supporting data. The number and variety of databases generated by federal agencies is impressive, but the variety of agencies involves means that databases vary in coverage, content, format, cost, frequency and accessibility.

State and local governments are also major sources of health-related data. State governments generate a certain amount of demographic data, with each state having a state data center for demographic projections. Vital statistics data can often be obtained in the most timely fashion at the state level, in fact. States vary, however, in the types and quality of data they generate. University data centers may also be involved in the processing of demographic data. Local governments may generate demographic data for use in various planning functions. City or county governments may produce population projections, while county health departments are responsible for the collection and dissemination of vital statistics data.

Professional Associations. Various associations within the healthcare industry represent another source of health-related data. Chief among these are the American Medical Association (and related medical specialty organizations) and the American Hospital Association. There are also other organizations of personnel (e.g., American Dental Association) and facilities (e.g., National Association for Home Care) that maintain databases on their members and on activities related to the organization's membership. These databases are typically developed for internal use but are increasingly being made available to the outside parties.

A number of organizations have been formed in recent years that focus specifically on health data, while others have established formal sections that deal with health data within their broader context. The National Association of Health Data Organizations (NAHDO), for example, brings together disparate parties from the public and private sectors who have an interest in health data. The National Association of County and City Health Officers (NACCHO) has become very active in terms of access to health data for local planning purposes. The Health Information and Management Systems Society (HIMSS) is one of the largest organizations that is addressing this issue as a collateral consideration to data management issues.

In recent years, many professional associations have made an increasing amount of information on their members available to the research and business communities. Not only do such organizations have an interest in exchanging information with related groups, but they also have recognized the revenue generation potential of such databases. Some of these databases include only basic information, while others offer a wealth of detail.

Private Organizations. Many private organizations (mostly not-for-profit) collect and/or disseminate health-related data. Voluntary health associations often compile, repackage and/or disseminate such data. The American Cancer Society, for example, distributes morbidity and mortality data as it relates to its areas of interest. Some organizations, like Planned Parenthood, may commission special studies on fertility or related issues and subsequently publish this information.

Many organizations repackage data collected elsewhere (e.g., from the Census Bureau or the National Center for Health Statistics) and present it within a specialized context. The Population Reference Bureau, a private not-for-profit organization, distributes population statistics in various forms, for example. Some, like the American Association of Retired Persons (AARP), not only compile and disseminate secondary data but are actively involved in primary data collection, as well as the sponsorship of numerous studies that include some form of data collection.

Commercial Data Vendors. Commercial data vendors represent a fourth category of sources of health-related databases. These organizations have emerged to fill

Box 4.5 Marketing research: Make or buy?

A major decision in any marketing research initiative involves the assignment of responsibility for the research function. The range of research options includes: performing all marketing research in-house using internal resources; totally outsourcing the research process; or utilizing a combination of internal and external resources. Another "compromise" approach might involve bringing in an outside consultant to coordinate the use of internal resources for the marketing research. Different healthcare organizations pursue different paths among these options. Nevertheless, at some point the choice "to make or buy" will come up, and the organization must decide whether or not to bring in an outside consultant and/or outsource the research function. To a certain extent, the corporate culture of the organization will influence its willingness to utilize such outside resources.

There are several advantages to carrying out the marketing research using in-house resources. Assuming that staff are already in place, the marketing effort will require a reassignment of responsibilities rather than developing marketing capabilities *de novo*. No additional costs would be expected besides the opportunity costs of diverting resources from other projects. Presumably, in-house staff are familiar with the organization's services and products as well as its organizational structure. Research processes may already be in place and a certain amount of data (particularly secondary data) may have already been compiled.

The benefits accrued from utilizing an outside resource include: access to expertise not readily available in house, experience with similar projects in other settings, and access to methodologies, data and other tools not commonly available. Importantly, the outside expert can offer an objectivity that is very difficult to achieve when one is too close to the problem.

There are disadvantages to using outside experts as well. They can be very expensive and a certain level of sophistication is required in order to negotiate a reasonable contract. (Note that there are no small costs involved in carrying out research activities in house, particularly if no dedicated function is already in place.) There may be situations in which such sensitive data are involved that outside access may be undesirable. Further, an outsider is an outsider and there may be aspects of the community or organization that are difficult to understand without having an insider's perspective. Ultimately, every organization will have to weigh the pluses and minuses of the two approaches.

One way to resolve the issue of whether to implement in house or bring in a consultant is to ask some basic questions. Is it cheaper to outsource the work than to do it ourselves? (This assumes that the organization has a realistic understanding of the true cost of conducting research using in-house staff.) Does it involve a type of expertise that is not available in house? Are

(continued)

> **Box 4.5** (continued)
>
> special data, software or equipment required whose purchase would not be practical for a one-time study? Is the issue being studied significantly controversial or sensitive as to demand the input of an objective outsider? On the other hand, is the information of such a confidential nature that it needs to be kept "in the family"? Finally, the one question that should be asked with *every* proposed project is: Does in-house staff really have the time and resources to conduct this project?

perceived gaps in the availability of various categories of health data. These include commercial data vendors that establish and maintain their own proprietary databases, as well as those that reprocess and/or repackage existing data. Vendors may maintain databases on nursing homes, urgent care centers, or other types of facilities and make this information available in a variety of forms. Also included in this group are the major data vendors (e.g., ESRI Business Information, Claritas) who do not necessarily create health-related databases but incorporate health-specific databases into their business database systems.

Because of the demand for health-related data, several commercial data vendors have added health data to their inventories, and a few health-specific data vendors have emerged. These vendors not only repackage existing data into more palatable form, but may develop their own proprietary databases.

The Internet. The Internet is already becoming a force with regard to health data. Although the focus at the time of this writing has been on consumer-oriented health information on the World Wide Web, data for use by health professionals is rapidly expanding. Bibliographical and text files are already becoming available, and some health care organizations are transferring patient data over the Internet. In the future, there is every reason to believe that data for marketing research will be widely available on the World Wide Web. (Box 4.5 discusses the relatively advantages of "making or buying" marketing data.)

Chapter 5
Marketing Planning

In marketing as in other endeavors, a well thought out plan of attack is essential. The actual marketing campaign is only launched after much of the marketing plan has been carried out. To a great extent the effectiveness of the initiative will reflect the quality of plan that is formulated. This chapter describes the steps involved in marketing planning and offers guidance on effective plan formulation.

Planning for Marketing

Marketing planning refers to *the development of a systematic process for promoting an organization, an idea or a product*. When marketing was previously described, the importance of the planning component was noted. Whether the targeted customer is the patient, the referring physician, the employer, the health plan, or any number of other possibilities, the marketing plan is built around someone's needs. Although a consideration of internal factors is often pertinent, the marketing plan focuses on the characteristics of the external market with the objective of influencing change in one or more of its characteristics.

As the term "planning" implies, the primary goal of the plan is to lay out a process for achieving a stated marketing goal. In addition to providing the "road map" for achieving the goal, the plan provides a basis for coordinating activities, marshalling resources, implementing tasks, and conducting evaluation of the initiative's effectiveness.

Nature of the Plan

The approach to marketing planning is going to vary depending on the focus of the initiative. In the case of a new organization or product, the intent is to create awareness, generate initial business, and establish a customer base. In the case of an existing

> **Box 5.1** Different levels of planning
>
> Marketing planning within a healthcare organization can take place at the following levels:
>
> * System-level or enterprise-wide marketing planning
> * Community-level marketing planning
> * Facility-level marketing planning
> * Product line marketing planning
> * Department-level marketing planning
> * Unit-level marketing planning

organization or product, the intent is to retain customers and enhance existing relationships. The plan should therefore reflect the particular situation faced by the marketer.

The scope of a marketing plan will reflect the complexity of the initiative being planned. The scope could range from the microlevel in which the marketing of a discrete event is being planned to the macrolevel at which the marketing direction for a mega health system is being charted. Of course, there are various levels of planning in between. (Box 5.1 indicates the different levels at which planning might occur.)

Most marketing plans are geared toward a lower level of operation. The typical marketing plan focuses on a particular service, program or even an event. A marketing plan developed to roll out a new service, office site or piece of equipment or a promotional plan for a series of patient education seminars would be fairly narrow in its scope and short-term in its duration (i.e., tactical). The long-term marketing plan for a large healthcare system would be much broader in scope and consider initiatives covering several years. Large scale marketing planning is less common but, when it occurs, it requires substantial resources.

Timeframe for Marketing Planning

Just as marketing plans vary in scope, they also display a range in terms of duration. The timeframe for most marketing plans is relatively narrow since the typical marketing initiative is short-term and involves a quick turnaround. Marketing planning for a one-time event might take place over a 3-month period culminating in the event for a total duration of no more than 4 months. On the other hand, an enterprise-wide marketing plan for an organization may easily cover 3–5 years in terms of its planned activities.

The Marketing Planning Process

Planning for Planning

The first step in any planning process involves identifying the mandate under which the planners are to operate. In other words: Why are we doing this? Who wants it done? The "why" of the marketing initiative is likely to color all subsequent activities and should be addressed early in the process.

Initial marketing planning activity involves identifying the key stakeholders, decision makers, and resource persons that must be taken into consideration. If the organization has an established marketing department, much of the initial background research may have already been completed, and the key players may be in place. However, in the case of a newly established marketing function or the marketing of an unfamiliar service, additional organizational effort is likely to be required.

The participants in the planning process should be drawn from a wide range of functional areas. In addition to marketing staff, there should be representatives from management, research, finance, human resources, information technology and clinical departments as appropriate. (See Box 5.2 for an overview of the composition of the planning team.)

The format for the planning process, the objectives of the process (but not the plan at this point), and such practical issues as the frequency of planning team meetings should be considered. Importantly, the purpose of the scheduled meetings – e.g.,

---

Box 5.2 Composition of the marketing planning team

The size and composition of the marketing planning team will depend on the nature and scope of the marketing initiative. Obviously, for an enterprise-wide plan the team will be larger and broader than for the planning of a specific event. For most planning purposes the following perspectives should be represented on the planning team:

- Marketing department staff
- Outside marketing resource (as appropriate)
- Public relations/communication staff (if separate)
- Administration
- Service line management staff (as appropriate)
- Research staff
- Health information management (medical records) staff
- Information technology staff
- Relevant clinical staff
- Finance department staff
- Relevant product-specific personnel

work sessions, progress reporting, decision making – must be specified. In addition to getting everyone on the "same page," the plan should indicate who is responsible for which tasks and when they should be performed.

Stating Assumptions

The stating of assumptions at the outset and throughout the planning process is critical. Certain assumptions can – and should – be made early in the planning process. Other assumptions will be developed as more information is collected and greater knowledge gained concerning the market, its healthcare needs, and available services. Assumptions might be initially stated with regard to the following issues:

- The organization
- The market
- The product
- The competition
- The reimbursement potential
- Resource availability

Initial Information Gathering

The effort devoted to initial data gathering will reflect the existing level of knowledge possessed by the marketing team. The data collection process begins with general background information on the organization, involving a review of any materials that have been prepared on the organization and on the particular product to be marketed. In addition to determining the attributes of the organization and/or its services, the marketer needs to determine the degree to which the organization or service is different from others and the extent of these differences.

This initial information gathering process should also reveal something about the history of the organization, service or product being marketed. The organization's "life history" will be instructive in developing a plan for its future, with the corporate culture exerting a strong influence on the marketing mindset.

An early step typically involves inventorying existing marketing resources and determining the extent to which current marketing activities relate to the proposed project. It is easy to overlook on-going marketing activities (especially if they are not labeled as such), but duplication of effort should be minimized. At the same time, the possibility of marketing activities operating at cross-purposes needs to be avoided.

The gathering of information serves, among other functions, as a means of testing the assumptions that have been stated. With the completion of additional research, it will be possible to review previously stated assumptions and revise them as appropriate. (Box 5.3 indicates some sources of background information.)

Box 5.3 Sources of background information
- Published documents about the organization
- Previously completed analyses (e.g., strategic plans, patient satisfaction studies)
- Reports filed (e.g., state health facility reports, CON applications)
- Unpublished documents (e.g., task force reports, retreat minutes)
- Independent market assessments
- Interviews with key informants

Information available on similar marketing initiatives in other markets can be helpful, especially if the initiative involves a product, market or approach with which the marketer has limited familiarity. The marketer should be able to incorporate information about marketing approaches that have and have not worked when similar organizations or services were being marketed in other contexts. (Additional information on marketing research is provided in Chapter 4.)

The Marketing Audit

The marketing planning process will typically involve an audit of both internal and external attributes. The internal audit, as the term implies, involves a review of internal systems and the information they can provide relative to the marketing effort. The external audit (or environmental assessment) examines conditions outside the walls of the organization relative to their implications for the marketing effort.

Internal audit. In performing the internal audit a number of different aspects of the organization should be examined. Some or all of the following aspects of the organization would be of interest at this point:

- Services/products descriptions
- Customer characteristics
- Utilization patterns
- Marketing arrangements
- Service delivery locations
- Referral relationships

The internal audit serves the purposes of telling us who we are, what we are doing and how well we're doing it. (The internal audit is discussed in more detail in Chapter 4.)

External audit. The external audit (or environmental assessment) typically begins with an examination of broad social, economic and political trends. National trends in demographics, lifestyles and attitudes are reviewed and their implications for consumer behavior in the targeted community considered.

Trends affecting the healthcare industry are analyzed as they relate to reimbursement patterns, changing organizational structures, the introduction of new treatment modalities and so forth. The political environment should be assessed along with developments in certificate-of-need requirements and other policies at the local level.

The analysis of the local market begins with the delineation of the market area and the profiling of the market area population. At a minimum, the analyst will examine the population in terms of age, sex, race/ethnicity, marital status/family structure, income and education. The demographic analysis may be accompanied by an assessment of the psychographic characteristics of the market area population.

The health status of the market area population can be examined in terms of fertility characteristics, morbidity levels as indicated by measures of incidence and prevalence for various health conditions, and mortality patterns that reveal the relationship between death and the size, composition, and distribution of the population.

Both formal and informal health behavior should be considered. Indicators of formal health behavior include hospital admissions, patient days, average length of stay, utilization of other facilities besides hospitals, physician office visits, visits to nonphysician practitioners, and drug utilization. Informal indicators of health behavior would include information on lifestyles, prevention activities, dietary patterns, and risky behaviors.

The external audit should involve some type of competitive analysis that determines the position of the organization within the market. We need to know who our competitors are, what their position in the market is, and what their presence means to us. The degree of detail involved in the competitive analysis depends on the nature of the organization and the type of marketing that is being initiated. (The external audit is discussed in more detail in Chapter 4.)

Setting Goals

The goal represents the generalized accomplishments that the organization would like to achieve through the marketing initiative. The goal or goals that are established in the marketing plan should reflect the information generated by means of the background research and be in keeping with the organization's mission statement. The goal may be narrow or broad in scope, depending on the nature of the marketing initiative.

A marketing goal should be a generalized statement that is limited in detail. It should be stated in a form such as: To establish Hospital X as the most visible facility in this market area, or to substantially increase the organization's market share among OB patients.

Marketers entering healthcare from other industries are likely to be surprised with the diffuseness of goals in healthcare. For many industries, the only possible goal is improvement in the bottom line. It is unfathomable that any initiative would be launched that did not have making money as its primary aim. This is clearly not the situation for many healthcare marketing initiatives, and this is why the organization's mission statement must be kept in mind when developing a marketing plan.

Determining Strategies

Once a marketing goal has been decided upon, a strategy must be selected. The strategy refers to the generalized approach that is to be taken in achieving the goal of the marketing initiative. Strategies set the tone for subsequent planning activities and in effect establish the parameters within which the marketer must operate. Ideally, the strategy employed for a marketing initiative will support the organization's mission statement and reflect the strategies embodied in the organization's strategic plan. The strategy could, for example, be framed in terms of an educational initiative, a public relations rather than an advertising approach, or a soft-sell versus a hard-sell approach, reflecting strategies established for the organization. (Strategy development is considered in more detail in Chapter 8.)

Setting Objectives

Having established a goal for the marketing initiative, the next step involves the formulation of objectives to support the attainment of that goal. Objectives refer to the specific mechanisms put into place for accomplishing marketing goals. Objectives should be clearly and concisely stated, and any concepts must be operationalizable and measurable. Objectives must also be time bound, with clear deadlines established for their accomplishment. Further, objectives must be amenable to evaluation. This is particularly critical since the success of the marketing plan should be measured by its success in achieving the stated objectives.

For every goal a number of objectives may be specified. Marketing objectives are stated in such terms as: The proportion of the general population for whom Hospital X is top of mind will be increased from 10 to 25% within 6 months (in support of the stated goal of making Hospital X top of mind in the community). The breadth of the goal will determine the number of objectives that are formulated.

Prioritizing Objectives

While all of the specified objectives may be considered important or even essential, it simply may not be feasible to pursue each of the objectives, or at least not all at the same time. Indeed, some objectives may potentially operate at cross-purposes with others, making it necessary to prioritize marketing efforts in favor of one or the other.

One approach that might be used for prioritizing the objectives of a marketing plan involves the traditional "four P's" of marketing: product, price, place and promotion. The decision could be made, for example, to focus on the product in the marketing initiative, at the expense of price, place and promotion. Thus, objectives that are most directly related to promoting the characteristics of the product would be emphasized. Or, it might be appropriate to capitalize on the price advantage of the product, thereby encouraging an emphasis on objectives that focus on the pricing dimension.

Any barriers to achieving the stated objectives of the organization should be identified and assessed at this point. While most barriers can be overcome, some barriers may end up being deal breakers. (Box 5.4 provides examples of issues to consider in establishing objectives.)

One other consideration at this point is the possibility of unanticipated consequences resulting from the meeting of any of the objectives. Although it may appear tedious, it is important to specify the likely consequences of pursuing each objective. This should involve a determination of both intended and unintended consequences. Too often the positive aspects of the situation are examined in isolation from the negative consequences that may result from the pursuit of the objective. These issues should also be considered in the formulation of assumptions.

Specifying Actions

The next step in the marketing planning process is the specification of the actions to be carried out. It is one thing to indicate what should be done, it is another to specify how it should be operationalized. For each of the objectives that have been identified a set of actions must be specified. These actions take a wide range of

---

Box 5.4 Issues in establishing objectives

There are a number of reasons why an ostensibly reasonable objective might be problematic. In accessing the appropriateness of an objective, the following issues should be considered:

- Ethical considerations
- Legal constraints
- Appropriateness and tastefulness
- Resonance with the target audience
- Service delivery issues
- Unintended consequences

forms, from assuring that postage is available to support a direct mail initiative to enlisting a celebrity spokesperson as a means of reaching an objective.

If the objective of a specialty practice is to raise awareness of its new sports medicine program, for example, a number of actions must be carried out. These may include: selecting an advertising agency, allocating funds for marketing, "packaging" the program, recruiting promotional spokespersons, and so forth. Many of these actions imply a certain sequence, and this is a point at which the original project plan might be further refined to specify the sequencing of the action steps.

The action steps developed for a marketing plan may be relatively standardized. It is likely that marketing initiatives are already underway, and this is an activity that is frequently carried out by the organization. A reasonable understanding of marketing resource requirements is likely to have been previously established, and there may be parties that already have responsibilities that would be directed toward the planning initiative. (Box 5.5 presents examples of goals, objectives and actions pursuant to a marketing plan.)

Box 5.5 Goals, objectives, and actions

The goals, objectives and actions for XYZ Healthcare might break out as follows:

Marketing goal
To establish XYZ as the premier general hospital in the minds of consumers in its market area.

Marketing objectives

1. Increase top-of-mind awareness of XYZ from 40% of consumers to 60% of consumers within 12 months.
2. Improve patient satisfaction ratings for XYZ patients from 80% excellent ratings to 90% excellent ratings within 12 months.
3. Increase the number of physicians regularly referring to XYZ by 25% over the next 12 months.

Sample marketing actions
For objective 1:

1. Develop an advertising campaign for local television
2. Increase XYZ event sponsorship from two events per year to four events.
3. Distribute an XYZ newsletter to all relevant members of the medical community.
4. Establish an interactive website featuring consumer-oriented information on XYZ's services.

Implementing the Marketing Plan

The payoff for the planning effort comes in the implementation of the plan. The planning process creates a road map that the marketer must use it to get where he wants to go. Marketing planners have an advantage in that the hand-off from planning to implementation is likely to be smoother than it is for other types of planning. Indeed, the same parties are likely to be involved in both activities.

In order to approach plan implementation systematically, it is important to include adequate detail in the project plan and develop an implementation matrix. The project plan systematically depicts the various steps in the planning process and specifies the sequence that they should follow. The project plan also indicates the relationships that exist between the various tasks and, importantly, the extent to which the completion of some tasks is a prerequisite for the accomplishment of others.

Project planning tools like Gantt charts help create a framework within which planners can work. Project management tools such as the program evaluation review technique (PERT) and the critical path method (CPM) offer useful aids for estimating the resources needed for clarifying the planning and control process. PERT involves dividing the total research project into its smallest component activities, determining the sequence in which these activities must be performed, attaching a time estimate for each activity, and presenting them in the form of a flow chart that allows a visual inspection of the overall process. These tools can be readily accessed today using computer software packages.

The implementation matrix should list every action called for by the plan, breaking each action down into tasks, if appropriate. For each action or task the responsible party should be identified, along with any secondary parties that should be involved in this activity. The matrix should indicate resource requirements (in terms of staff time, money and other requirements). The start and end dates for this activity should be identified. Any prerequisites for accomplishing this task should be identified at the outset (and factored into the project plan). Finally, some benchmark should probably be stated that allows the planning team to determine when the activity has been completed

The resource requirements from the implementation matrix should be combined to determine total project resource requirements. Once identified, the extent of the requirements may have to be addressed in relation to available funds and any other fiscal constraints.

There are well-established techniques for implementing a marketing plan. The implementation plan can focus on a traditional media campaign with heavy advertising or it might emphasize direct marketing. On the other hand, perhaps internal marketing is the most efficacious approach to take. Or, the situation may call for business-to-business marketing. If a media approach is chosen, the type of media to be utilized becomes an issue for the implementation plan. The techniques utilized will be dictated by the nature of the marketing initiative. (See Box 5.6 for an example of an implementation matrix.)

Box 5.6 Sample excerpt from an implementation matrix

Task/ Subtask	Description	Primary Responsibility	Secondary Responsibility	Resource Requirements	Pre-requisites	Start Date	End Date
Market research							
Market profile	On-going review of target area demographics, lifestyles, socioeconomic status, etc.	Research Director				3/1/2005	4/15/2005
Demand estimates	On-going analysis of consumer demand for health services	Research Director				3/15/2005	4/15/2005
Employer analysis	Initial inventory of potential downtown employers for marketing	Research Director	Communications Director			3/15/2005	4/15/2005
Employer targeting	Identification of downtown employers for targeting	Communications Director				5/1/2005	On-going
Partner needs assessment	On-going solicitation of feedback from partners and business clients	Research Director	Communications Director			4/15/2005	5/1/505
Marketing evaluation	Development of evaluation plan, including pretest and post-test of the target audience(s)	Research Director		Survey capabilities	Baseline data collection	4/1/2005	On-going
Client satisfaction	Development/automation of client satisfaction instrument	Research Director			Interview form/web enablement	6/1/2005	On-going
Brand development							
Brand conceptualization	Determine the nature of the H of H brand and specify the components of its brand identity.	All				4/15/2005	5/15/2005
Brand copy	In coordination with copy development for other media, prepare copy for brand promotion	Copy Writer				6/1/2005	6/15/2005

Product branding opportunities	Identify goods and services that it makes sense to try to brand	All	5/15/2005	6/15/2005
Branding partner identification	Identify potential partners for the development of branded products	Media Consultant	6/1/2005	7/1/2005
Brand materials preparation	Design and produce materials to support the brand	Copy Writer	6/15/2005	7/15/2005
Corporate (collateral) materials				
Copy preparation	Prepare copy for use in preparation of collateral materials and other promotional activities	Copy Writer	4/1/2005	4/15/2005
Finalize brochure	Revise/finalize brochure for multipurpose distribution	Communications Director	5/1/2005	5/1/2005
Print brochure	Identify and utilize printing resource (preferably from among partners)	Communications Director	5/15/2005	6/1/2005
Letterhead	Prepare letterhead reflecting logo and other brand images	Communications Director	6/1/2005	6/15/2005
Business cards	Revise business cards with new brand image	Communications Director	6/1/2005	6/15/2005
Website content	Modify/incorporate general promotion copy into Website	All	5/1/2005	6/15/2005
Posters	Design/produce posters for strategic placement	Copy Writer	5/15/2005	6/15/2005
Media kit	Design/develop a multipurpose media ket	Copy Writer	6/1/2005	6/15/2005

Box 5.7 Marketing plan checklist

This checklist provides a useful guide for determining if all steps in the marketing plan have been performed:
— Specify the marketing "problem"
— Identify relevant participants
— Organize the planning effort
— Compile background information
— State assumptions
— Conduct additional research
— Perform internal audit
— Perform external audit
— Specify the marketing goal
— Formulate the marketing strategy
— Specify the marketing objectives
— Refine and prioritize objectives
— Develop the implementation matrix
— Implement the plan
— Evaluate campaign
— Revise the plan (as appropriate)

Evaluating the Marketing Plan

The evaluation of the marketing plan should be top of mind on the first day of the process and, in fact, should be built into the process itself. It should involve on-going monitoring of the process, involving benchmarks and/or milestones for assessment along the way. While the evaluation process is important for all types of planning processes, it is particularly important in marketing planning. Managing the marketing plan is essential to managing the marketing process.

Evaluation techniques focus to two types of analysis: process (or formative) analysis and outcome (or summative) analysis. Both of these have a role to play in the project, although outcome evaluation is particularly important for marketing initiatives. Process evaluation should assess the efficiency of the marketing effort. For the outcome evaluation, changes in image or sales volume must be measured, with the success of the project calculated in relatively precise terms. (Evaluation techniques are discussed in more detail in Chapter 12. Box 5.7 presents a marketing planning checklist.)

Chapter 6
Healthcare Products and Customers

The first concerns of any marketer are the nature of the product being marketed and the characteristics of the customers to whom it is being marketed. This chapter addresses the issues involved in defining and packaging healthcare products and determining the characteristics of potential customers. Different ways of segmenting the target audience are presented.

Products and Customers

Marketing focuses on the link between two key elements: a product and a market – and the primary goal of the marketer is to connect the two. The first challenge for healthcare marketers is to define the "product" to be promoted. Any marketer – particularly one from another industry – is going to ask right off: What are we selling? Our tendency is to say something high-minded like "health" or "effective outcomes" or "quality of life." Health professional often must be assested in define their products.

The second question that needs to be asked is: Who are we selling it to? This may be an obvious question but, remember, the healthcare industry – particularly the hospital component – has historically tried to sell all things to all people. As the industry matured, healthcare executives realized that they could not sell everything to everyone, and the specific market (or markets) for the organization's services needed to be identified. Obviously, the wider the appeal of the service (e.g., general inpatient care) the broader the market; the more specific the service (e.g., hair transplantation) the narrower the market. Either way, the marketer must be able to target the audience that is most likely to need the service in question. (More about targeting audiences is presented later in the chapter.)

The Product Mix

An organization's "product mix" refers to the combination of goods, services and even ideas that it offers. Much of what healthcare organizations promote takes the form of ideas, intangible concepts that are intended to convey a perception to the consumer. The organization's image is an idea that is likely to be conveyed through marketing activities. The organization may want to promote the perception of quality care, professionalism, value or some other subjective attribute. The development of a brand, for example, would involve the marketing of an idea. The intent here, of course, is to establish the organization at the top of the consumers mind on the assumption that familiarity will breed utilization.

Most healthcare organizations offer one or more less conceptual products to their customers. Further, a major hospital will offer hundreds if not thousands of different procedures. In addition, it offers a variety of goods (in the form of drugs, supplies and equipment) that are charged to the customer. The hospital may manage gift shops and provide food service to its customers as well.

Healthcare providers are generally more concerned with the promotion of services than goods. The nature of services in healthcare, however, is often difficult to describe. While a physician might break services down by procedure code (e.g., CPT code), few services truly stand alone. The group of services that constitutes a particular surgical procedure, for example, may be "bundled" together in the consumer's mind. While clinicians (and their billing clerks) may see them as discrete services, the patient perceives of them as a complex of services related to a heart attack, diabetes management, or cancer treatment. (Box 6.1 discusses issues in defining healthcare products.)

The marketer's task is to conceptualize the product and "package" it in a manner appropriate for marketing purposes. Ultimately, however, the marketer has to conceive of the service in a manner to which the consumer can relate. (Box 6.2 describes service lines as a means of packing health services.)

Elective and Nonelective Procedures

An important distinction among healthcare products is between elective procedures and nonelective procedures. Nonelective procedures are those that are considered medically necessary. Elective procedures are those that patients voluntarily choose to obtain. Nonelective procedures include life-saving measures, although medically necessary services do not always deal with life-threatening conditions. Elective procedures include, for example, nontherapeutic abortions, laser eye surgery, facelifts and hair transplants. Some joint surgery (e.g., for tennis elbow) might not be considered medically necessary and thus be classified as elective.

While some elective and nonelective procedures might be marketed in much the same manner, there are significant differences to note. For one thing, the decision maker is likely to be different. Nonelective surgery is generally "prescribed" by a medical practitioner and, being medically necessary, is generally covered by health

Box 6.1 Defining the "product"

The marketing process might be thought to begin with an accurate definition of the product and the specification of its characteristics. The marketer must know what he is selling, whether it is a good, a service, an organization or an idea. The questions below should be asked to determine the nature of the product to be marketed:

- How can the product be described in a sentence or two?
- Will all relevant parties understand that description?
- What are the products defining characteristics?
- How can this product be differentiated from other products being offered and from competitors' products?
- What is the current position of this product in the market?
- What is the history of this product in this market?
- What "space" in the market does it occupy or seek to occupy?
- What past or existing marketing activities have been carried out vis-à-vis this product?
- At what stage of the product life cycle can the product be considered to be?
- What is the perception of this product within the target population?
- What is the level of customer acceptance of/satisfaction with this product?
- Are there examples of successful promotional efforts available for this product?
- How well is the organization prepared to respond to a successful marketing initiative for this product?

Box 6.2 The service line

In the 1980s, following the lead of other industries, healthcare organizations began to develop service lines. Many industries think in terms of product lines, but in healthcare service lines seems to be more appropriate. The establishment of service lines involves organizing the programs of the hospital into vertical groupings focused on a particular clinical area. Categories of services often grouped as service lines include women's services, cancer services, cardiology, orthopedics, and pediatrics. Each service line is considered semi-autonomous and has responsibility for the vertical integration of its services. Thus, the service line administrator has broad control over the range of activities (including marketing) that supports the service line.

Some observers contend that services lines represent little more than the packaging of services for marketing purposes. While there are certainly cases in which the service line is more in the packaging than in the substance, in most cases a certain level of reorganization occurs around the specific clinical area. The use of the service line approach in healthcare remains controversial and tits merits are still being discussed today. Regardless of the merits of this approach, service line management invariably includes a significant marketing component.

insurance plans. The decision to undergo an elective procedure is generally made by the patient, perhaps with the advice of a medical practitioner. Because of its elective nature, these procedures are typically *not* covered by insurance.

The distinction between elective and nonelective procedures dictates different appeals to the respective set of consumers. For nonelective procedures, the demand cannot be easily influenced by marketing. Thus, the emphasis must be on influencing the choice of provider when a condition arises. A hospital seeking patients for nonelective procedures may focus its marketing on admitting and referring physicians since these are the parties likely to make decisions with regard to hospitalization.

Elective services are likely to be marketed like other consumer products. Providers of elective services are much more prone to advertise their services and often compete on the same basis as providers of other types of services. Thus, eye surgeons and plastic surgeons may advertise their low prices, convenient locations, and efficient customer service. In addition, it may actually be possible to *create* demand for these services. By introducing a new cosmetic surgery procedure (e.g., botox), a market may be created where none existed before.

Packaging the Product

Health professionals typically do not think in terms of "packaging" their services. Most feel that they are offering a standard product that is little different from those of other providers. One gall bladder surgery is much like any other gall bladder surgery. To health professionals, packaging sounds like something you do with cereal or candy bars.

Of course, not all health professionals view packaging this way. There are numerous examples of providers offering elective services that require differentiation and aggressive promotion. Ophthalmic surgeons actively promote their latest technology, and cosmetic surgeons attempt to demonstrate their superior skills. Services that must be paid for out of pocket – and where the end-user is likely to make the purchase decision – have long emphasized packaging as a prerequisite for marketing.

Packaging occurs anytime a healthcare organization designs a service in a way that it will appeal to the target audience. This may be as simple as giving the service a catchy name (e.g., "The New You" for a weight management program). Or it may be as complex as creating a distinct brand around a particular service.

In an environment where many services are standardized, it may be the packaging that distinguishes one product from another. Where possible the package should be enhanced to make it more distinctive and appealing. Free child-birth classes provided to those who plan to deliver their babies at the hospital may enhance the package. Or, creating a home-like environment in the birthing center might similarly contribute to the packaging.

The other part of packaging is the presentation. The service might be presented as "state-of-the-art," "patient-friendly," or delivered with a "touch of love."

Describing the product in this manner helps set it apart from similar, hopefully less appealing, services. Presentation without substance, however, can do more harm than good, so it is important that the organization be able to provide the service in the manner described. (Box 6.3 describes the emergence of retail medicine where effective packaging is essential.)

Box 6.3 The emergence of "retail" medicine

The concept of "retail medicine," or healthcare that is available to consumers outside of a traditional institutional setting, is coming to occupy a new niche in the elective outpatient marketplace. While there is no definitive estimate of the number of retail medicine centers in the United States, established outpatient facilities are cashing in on the trend and diversifying their existing menu of diagnostic and surgical services.

For example, we've seen the development of the "one-stop retail center" for elective procedures. Centers are being established for body imaging, heart scanning, lung screening and virtual colonoscopy. The setting for screening and imaging varies from outpatient radiology clinics to hospital campuses to wellness centers. Radiology practices are also expanding the use of cutting-edge diagnostic services to the large group of individuals who are currently without symptoms but concerned about prevention.

Aging baby boomers – the vast majority of the individuals who consume retail medicine – are more concerned about their health than any previous generation, and they are driving a lot of the interest in retail marketing. One of the most sought-after components of the retail medicine trend is the full-body scan, which medical entrepreneurs say will reveal abnormalities in the body that can be addressed before they have a chance to become life threatening. Computerized tomography (CT) scans promise to detect latent signs of conditions ranging from tumors to gallstones, clogged arteries to cancer.

Retail medicine often emphasizes prevention, an aspect of care that is largely ignored by hospitals and physician practices. The owners of screening centers are giving the public what they inherently understand – that prevention is better than a cure and early detection is the key to successful preventive strategies. Also included as examples of retail medicine are the variety of fitness and wellness programs that healthcare organizations are offering to the general public.

There has also been a trend toward the retailing of various goods through physicians' offices. Cardiologists may offer resources like books, videos and audiotapes on heart health and rehabilitation for purchase by their patients. Obstetricians and pediatricians might sell resource materials on childbirth and parenting. Dermatologists may offer a range of products for skin care, sun protection, and hair growth. Today, a variety of different practitioners vend nutritional supplements and vitamins as a sideline to their practices.

Healthcare Customers

The Variety of Healthcare Customers

While we may think in terms of individuals as consumers of healthcare, health professionals and facilities are also major consumers of goods and services in the healthcare arena. Indeed, the end-user for a service (e.g., a patient) may not even be considered the "customer" in many cases. And so, as seen in Chapter 2, the customer may go by a variety of names.

Even "patients" fall into a variety of different categories, each with specific needs. While some patients may require life-saving services, the typical healthcare customer is in need of "routine" healthcare. These include the typical person who presents himself for treatment at a doctor's office, clinic, or therapy center. This category constitutes the bulk of episodes for those requiring formal healthcare. A third category would include consumers who desire elective health services. As noted earlier, these would include products and/or services that are not considered medically necessary and are not likely to be covered by insurance.

There is also the major category of consumers who are involved in self care. Research has indicated that the amount of self care is much greater than previously thought and that accessing the formal healthcare system typically occurs *after* other options have been exhausted. Thus, it is typical for symptomatic individuals to self diagnose and self medicate, employing the wide range of "do-it-yourself" healthcare products that have become available. Pharmacy shelves have become stocked with a variety of products and devices for home testing and treatment, and the Internet has expanded the availability of such products.

For these and other reasons, a number of different terms are being applied today to the purchasers and/or end-users of healthcare goods and services. At the practitioner level, the term "patient" is giving way to other terms that more clearly reflect the contemporary healthcare environment. (See Chapter 2 for a discussion of the various "labels" attached to customers. Box 6.4 presents the contrasting characteristics of healthcare consumers and other types of consumers.)

Professional and Institutional Customers

As noted above, the end-user of healthcare goods and services represents only one of the customer categories found in healthcare. Much of the consumption of goods and services is carried out by health professionals and healthcare institutions. Although the *physician* is thought of as a provider of services rather than a consumer of them, physician practices actually represent a major customer for many goods and services. Hospitals solicit physicians to join their medical staffs (and service them once they join). Provider networks and health plans solicit the participation of physicians and other clinicians. Nursing homes,

Box 6.4 Healthcare consumers versus other consumers

Consumers of Health Services	Consumers of Other Services
Seldom determine their need for services	Usually determine their need for services
Seldom the ultimate decision maker	Usually the ultimate decision maker
Often subjective basis for decision	Usually objective basis for decision
Seldom has knowledge of the price	Always has knowledge of the dup price
Seldom makes decision based on price	Usually makes decision based on price
Cost mostly covered by a third party	Cost virtually never covered by a third party
Usually nondiscretionary purchase	Usually discretionary purchase
Usually requires a professional referral	Almost never requires a professional referral
Limited choice among available options	No limit to choice among available options
Limited knowledge of service attributes	Significant knowledge of service attributes
Limited ability to judge quality of service	Usually able to judge quality of service
Limited ability to evaluate outcome	Able to evaluate outcome
Little recourse for unfavorable outcome	Ample recourse for unfavorable outcome
Seldom the ultimate target for marketing	Always the ultimate target for marketing
Not susceptible to standard marketing techniques	Susceptible to standard marketing techniques

home health agencies, and hospices may depend on them for their referrals. Many physicians depend on referrals from other physicians and those referring physicians represent customers.

Physicians also serve as customers for a variety of organizations providing support services. These include billing and collection services, utilization review companies, medical supply distributors, biomedical equipment companies, and biohazard management companies. Physicians are also customers for information technology vendors who sell and/or service practice management systems, imaging systems, and/or electronic patient records.

Physicians have traditionally been the primary customer for pharmaceutical companies. The extent to which pharmaceutical companies will go to acquire physician loyalty to their drug lines is legendary. In fact, the sales and promotions efforts of pharmaceutical companies toward physicians became so intense that Congress ultimately had to pass regulations restricting attempts by pharmaceutical companies to influence the prescribing practices of physicians.

Other clinicians are customers for many of the same goods and services as physicians. Dentists, optometrists, podiatrists, chiropractors, mental health counselors and other independent practitioners have many of the same needs as physicians and are cultivated by similar marketing entities. These providers require supplies, equipment, billing and collections, information technology and other services just as physicians do.

Hospitals and other healthcare institutional settings have a wide-range of health-related requirements as well as the normal needs that any large organization must address. Like physicians, they require medical supplies and biomedical equipment. More so than physicians, they require durable medical equipment such as wheelchairs and hospital beds. They are customers for a wide range of support services, from billing and collections to physician recruitment to marketing. By virtue of providing food service, gift shops, and parking services, hospitals are customers for a wide variety of non–health-related goods and services. Hospitals and other healthcare facilities are heavy consumers of information technology and are major customers for IT venders and consultants.

Major *employers* represent customers for health plans, managed care plans, providers and provider networks. Most health plans are employer-based, and competing health plans seek to contract with employers for the management of their employees' health. Individual providers may seek to contract with employers that are self-insured or otherwise open to negotiated services. Employers are also customers for a variety of direct services from providers. These include a wide range of occupational health services, employee assistance programs, fitness center programs, and various other services that providers might market directly to employers.

Other "Customers"

Like organizations in other industries, healthcare organizations have various "internal" customers. Chief among these are their *employees*. Any organization must consider its associates as customers, and healthcare organizations have, unfortunately, not been in the forefront in this regard. It is important to continuously market the mission, goals and objectives of the organization to these internal customers and to regularly solicit their input. (See Box 6.5 for a discussion of employees as customers.)

Another internal customer would be the organization's *board of directors*. In most organizations the board of directors is charged with setting the direction of the organization and monitoring its progress. This body typically plays a critical role in

Box 6.5 Employees are customers too

Internal marketing refers to efforts by a service provider to effectively train and motivate its customer-contact employees and all the supporting service people to work as a team to promote the organization and improve customer satisfaction. Internal marketing aims to ensure that everybody within an organization is committed to its mission and is working towards the achievement of the organization's objectives. It recognizes that people who work together stand in exactly the same relationships to each other as do customers and suppliers.

In the absence of internal marketing, employees don't know what services are offered, what those in other departments are doing, or how they fit into the overall picture. They lose sight of the organization's mission and become focused on isolated tasks rather than the big picture. All this is bad news for the customer, the employee and the organization.

Effective internal marketing redefines employees as valued customers. The rationale is that anticipating, identifying and satisfying employee needs will lead to greater commitment. This in turn will allow the organization to improve the quality of service to its external customers. Although internal marketing efforts will necessarily involve a number of departments, the marketing department is a logical focal point to begin. Presumably the marketing department has knowledge about the organization's overall strategy, an appreciation of external customers needs, the expertise to deploy the appropriate tools with regard to internal customers, and the budgets and financial resources to do the job. Internal marketing begins with communication, and communication, of course, is the primary responsibility of the marketing staff.

Investment in internal efforts has always been a paltry fraction of most marketers' budgets, and this is probably more true of healthcare than other industries. But the process of internal marketing requires a great deal of training in order to instill the requisite knowledge and assure that all employees are on the same page. Companies that are frantically trying to boost revenues and cut costs may not see why they should spend money on their employees. Missing the point that these are the very people who ultimately deliver the brand promises the company makes. Internal marketing can also serve as an important implementation tool. It aids communication and helps the organization overcome resistance to change. It serves to involve all staff in new initiatives and strategies

There is nothing magic about internal marketing; in fact, most of it involves the application of common sense. Among the most common features of internal marketing programs are meetings. Special events, company anniversary celebrations, appreciation dinners, brown bag lunches, off-site/satellite offices visits, internal newsletters, bulletin boards, e-mail newsletters, intranets, and broadcast e-mails. It should be remembered, however, that internal marketing starts with new employee orientation and should be continuously reinforced through on-going training.

Any internal marketing initiative starts (and finishes) with top management. Senior administrators must be committed to the effort and be active players in the establishment and reinforcement of an appropriate corporate culture. They must also assure that adequate resources are available to support the internal marketing effort.

the operation of the organization and should be considered an important customer by the staff.

There are other "secondary" customers that should be considered as well. One of these is the *general public*. Most provider organizations and many other types of organizations in healthcare must maintain a positive public image. Not only is it important to create and sustain corporate goodwill, but it may be necessary to demonstrate at some point that the organization is a good community citizen and, in the case of a not-for-profit organization, that it deserves to retain its tax-exempt status.

Another customer for healthcare organizations is the *media*. The media require cultivation in order to assure that the organization's story is told and told in the right manner. Indeed, long before hospitals and other healthcare organizations had formal marketing functions, they had public relations departments to deal with the media.

For many healthcare organizations, one or more branches of *government* represent customers. Health facilities and health professions are regulated by government agencies and often maintain separate government relations offices. If the organization is not-for-profit, its tax-exempt status depends on maintaining good relationships with the appropriate government agencies. In areas where certificate-of-need requirements exist, healthcare organizations must maintain relationships with the appropriate agencies.

Prioritizing Customers

Given the wide range of customer types (and the variety of gatekeepers, referral agents, and decision makers), it may be difficult to know where to best focus the marketing effort. Should the bulk of the effort be directed toward the end-user or toward the party who will be making the decision or to the entity that is paying for the service? Alternatively, how does one allocate scarce resources among such a variety of options?

In this situation, as with much of marketing, the answer is determined by the situation. Marketing research can be used to determine who – end-user, decision maker, payer – represents the most logical target for the marketing effort. For services that depend heavily on referrals, there is little benefit in cultivating those who are not referral agents (even if they are using the services). On the other hand, for a service that is elective in nature it doesn't make sense to target anyone beside the end-user. (Of course, an exception might be the rare elective procedure for which someone besides the end-user – e.g., caretaker, parent – makes the decision.) If the customer's health plan restricts them to a particular healthcare facility, there may be little that can be done to influence the process. (However, if it is *your* health facility they must use, you can make sure that they have a positive experience.)

The situation may not always be clear-cut. With a general medical practice or a hospital, customers may arrive at the door through a variety of paths. Patients

Box 6.6 Prioritizing the marketing effort

- How did the customer find out about our services?
- Who made the decision for the customer to contact us?
- How much of a role did the end-user play in choosing our services?
- Was a "formal" referral involved (i.e., from a physician or other referral agent)?
- Was the customer channeled to our services through a health plan or employer?
- Are caregivers, parents/guardians, or other third-parties likely to be involved in decision making?
- Can marketing be employed to influence the observed process?
- If so, where can marketing be used to most effectively to influence utilization decisions?
- Are different marketing approaches necessary to address all of the parties involved?

may be self-referred or, in the case of the hospital, choose a particular emergency room. They may be referred by a physician or other clinician or even by some other type of referral agent (e.g., social service agency, discharge danner). They may be channeled to the organization by a health plan or managed care organization. Marketing research should indicate which patients originate in what manner. (Box 6.6 indicates some question that might be asked with regard to prioritizing your marketing effort.)

Once customers have been prioritized from a marketing perspective, decisions still have to be made with regard to the allocation of resources. Should virtually all resources be focused on the target audience that promises the most return or should all potential sources of customers be allocated *some* resources? Again, the answer is going to vary with the situation and here marketing research comes into play.

Consumer Attitudes

"Attitude" refers to a position an individual has adopted in response to a theory, belief, object, event, or another person. It establishes a relatively consistent, acquired predisposition to behave in a certain way in response to a given object. When "consumer attitudes" are considered in healthcare, they typically refer to the attitudes that influence the preferences, expectations, and behaviors of the end-user or purchaser of health services. Thus, attitudes held by consumers toward the healthcare system in general, physicians, particular facilities, certain treatments and so forth are thought to color the consumer decision-making process. Consumers' willingness to utilize urgent care centers rather than emergency rooms, health maintenance organizations rather than traditional health plans, and chiropractors rather than orthopedic surgeons may be a function of the attitudes they hold.

Attitudes are not restricted to the consumers of health services, and physicians and other health professionals also bring attitudes to the situation. The attitudes of physicians, for example, have been documented to have an impact on the likelihood of a malpractice suit being filed. Even organizations may be predisposed to certain attitudes, as in the case of healthcare organizations that are prejudiced against the use of consultants or tailor their service offerings to reflect the organization's religious underpinnings. Attitudes within the organization typically reflect that organization's corporate culture.

Although patterns of consumer attitudes in U.S. society tend to be complex, it is clear that a new orientation is occurring with regard to healthcare. For the most part, today's consumer is much more knowledgeable about the healthcare system, much more open to innovative approaches, and much more intent on playing an active role in the diagnostic, therapeutic and health maintenance processes.

These new attitudes are concentrated among the under-50 population and among certain demographically distinct groups. The movement toward gaining control of one's health has been spearheaded by the baby boom cohort that is now beginning to face the chronic conditions associated with "middle age." This is the population that has been responsible for the success of health maintenance organizations, urgent care centers and birthing centers. This is the group that has been influential in limiting the discretion and control of physicians and hospitals. This cohort has also provided the impetus for the rise of "alternative therapy" as a competitor for mainstream allopathic medicine.

The approach to healthcare favored by the baby boom population is more patient centered than the traditional approach and is more likely to emphasize the nonmedical aspects of healthcare. In general, baby boomers are less trusting of professionals and institutions and are control oriented to the point of stubbornness. This group is more self-reliant than previous post-WWII generations and places greater value on self-care and home care. It is both outcomes oriented and cost sensitive. It is a generation that prides itself in getting results and extracting value for its expenditures. While this cohort began influencing the healthcare system by "voting with its feet" during the 1980s, its members are increasingly in the positions of power that allow them to influence the reshaping the healthcare landscape.

To a certain extent, these new attitudes toward healthcare reflect the rise of consumerism across the societal spectum. *Customers* (as opposed to *patients*) expect to receive adequate information, participate in decisions that directly affect them, and receive the best possible care. Customers want to receive their healthcare close to their homes, with minimal interruption to their family life and work schedules. They also want to maximize the value that they receive for their healthcare expenditures. (Box 6.7 discusses some of the factors that drive consumer decision making.)

Box 6.7 What do healthcare consumers really want?

The nature of the healthcare consumer has been changing and along with that what they consider important in health services. Although it is difficult to generalize, contemporary healthcare consumers are likely to have an interest in the following service attributes:

- Quality
- Value
- Convenience
- Personal care
- Consistency
- Open communication
- Reliability
- Consideration of their time
- Streamlined billing
- Therapeutic environments
- Treatment options

Segmenting Healthcare Customers

Once healthcare moved away from mass marketing as a means of cultivating consumers, it began to adopt a more targeted approach based on market segmentation. Market segmentation, long utilized in other industries, is used to identify specific segments of the population that are subsequently singled out for targeted attention.

Not every subgroup within a population qualifies as a target market, and there are certain rules of thumb that help marketers identify a meaningful market segment. A viable market segment should be *measurable* in that accurate and complete information on customer characteristics can be acquired in a cost-effective manner. It should be *accessible* in that it is possible to communicate effectively with the chosen segment using standard marketing methods. It should be *substantial* enough to support dedicated marketing activity. And a segment should be *meaningful* in that it includes consumers who have attributes relevant to the aims of the marketer. A final consideration in healthcare is that a viable market segment should also evidence a desire for the product and have the ability to pay for care.

Market segmentation can take a number of different forms and some of the more common are describe below.

Demographic segmentation. Market segmentation on the basis of demographics is the best known of the approaches to identifying target markets. The links between demographic characteristics and health status, health-related attitudes, and health behavior have been well established. For this reason, demographic segmentation is always an early task in any marketing planning process, with demographically distinct subgroups defined relative to various goods and services.

Geographic segmentation. An understanding of the spatial distribution of the target market has become increasingly important as healthcare has become more consumer driven. One of the implications of this trend has been the increased emphasis on the appropriate location of health facilities. The market-driven approach to health services has demanded that healthcare organizations take their services to the population, and the major purchasers of health services are insisting on convenient locations for their enrollees. Knowledge of the manner in which the population is distributed within the service area and the linkage between geographic segmentation and other forms of segmentation is critical for the development of a marketing plan.

Psychographic segmentation. For many types of goods and services an understanding of the psychographic or lifestyle characteristics of the target population is essential. The lifestyle clusters that can be identified for a population often transcend (or at least complement) its demographic characteristics. Most importantly, psychographic traits can be linked to the attitudes, perceptions and expectations of the target population, as well as to the propensity to purchase various services and products. While psychographic analysis in healthcare has lagged behind its use in other industries, health professionals are finding an increasing number of applications for this approach, and growing amounts of healthcare data are being incorporated into psychographic segmentation systems.

Usage segmentation. A common form of segmentation long used by marketers is now being applied to healthcare. The market area population can be divided into categories based on the extent of use of a particular service. In the case of urgent care clinic usage, for example, the population can be divided into heavy users, moderate users, occasional users and nonusers. This approach can be applied to a wide range of services, of course, but may have its most important applications when elective goods and services are under consideration. This information provides a basis for subsequent marketing planning that can be tailored differently, for example, for existing loyal customers and noncustomers. The willingness of individuals to use certain services, especially elective procedures, often reflects the extent to which they fall into the category of "adopters." (See Box 6.8 for a discussion of adoption process for new healthcare services.)

Payor segmentation. A form of market segmentation unique to healthcare involves targeting population groups on the basis of their payor categories. The existence of insurance coverage and the type of coverage available are major considerations in the marketing of most health services. Further, health plans cover some services and not others, and this becomes an important consideration in marketing. For elective services that are paid for out of pocket, a targeted marketing approach is typically required. The payor mix of the market area population has now come to be one of the first considerations in profiling target populations.

Box 6.8 "Adopters" of innovative health services

Healthcare consumers vary significantly in terms of their willingness to adopt new healthcare modalities. As a result, marketers have studied the process through which individuals come to adopt a new procedure or therapeutic modality from first hearing about the innovation to final adoption. Various studies have found that the population can be subdivided into the categories of innovators, early adopters, early majority, late majority, and laggards.

Innovators represent on average the first 2.5% of all those who adopt. They are eager to try new ideas and products almost as an obsession. They have higher incomes, are better educated, and are more active outside their community than noninnovators. They are less reliant on group norms, more self confident, and more likely to obtain their information from scientific sources and experts.

Early adapters represent on average the next 13.5% to adopt product, adopting early in the product's life cycle. They are much more reliant on group norms and values than innovators, and are much more oriented to the local community than the innovators who have a more cosmopolitan outlook. Early adopters are more likely to be opinion leaders because of their closer affiliation to groups. They are regarded as the most important segment for determining whether a new product will be successful due to their personal influence on others.

The *early majority* represents the next 34% to adopt. They will deliberate more carefully before adopting a new product, collecting more information and evaluating more options than will the early adopters. Therefore, the process of adoption takes longer. They are an important link in the diffusion process as they are positioned between the earlier and later adopters.

The *late majority* represents the next 34% to adopt. They are described as skeptical, and they adopt because most of their friends have already done so. Since they rely on group norms, adoption is the result of the pressure to conform. They tend to be older, with below average income and education, relying primarily on word-of-mouth communication rather than the mass media.

Laggards represent the final 16% to adopt. They are similar to innovators in not relying on the norms of the group. They are independent because they are tradition-bound, with decisions made in terms of the past. By the time they adopt an innovation, it has probably been superseded by something else. Laggards have the lowest socioeconomic status.

Healthcare marketers can improve their effectiveness by determining the point at which their goods and services are in the product life cycle and using this information to target the components of the consumer population that are most likely to adopt the product. Marketing efforts can be directed toward those most likely to adopt a new service.

Source: Assael, Henry (1992). *Consumer Behavior and Marketing Action.* Mason, OH: Southwestern.

Benefit segmentation. Different people buy the same or similar products for different reasons. Benefit segmentation is based on the idea consumers can be grouped according to the principal benefit sought. The benefits that consumers consider when making a purchase decision related to a given good or service include such product attributes as quality, convenience, value, and ease of access. In an increasingly consumer-driven environment, benefit segmentation requires special attention.

Chapter 7
Paying the Marketing Freight

Managing the financial aspects of marketing is often a neglected function. Marketers are not accountants, and bulldogging a budget is not nearly as exciting as developing award-winning ad campaigns. In this chapter the resources necessary to support various forms of marketing are described and practical information provided on getting the most for the marketing investment. Guidance is provided on how to turn marketing from a cost center into a contributor to the organization's bottom line.

Marketing "Sticker Shock"

Whenever the topic of marketing comes up, the first thing that comes to mind for a healthcare executive is often the cost. Since healthcare administrators have historically had a poor understanding of the financial side of marketing, they often suffer from "sticker shock" when they are told what a marketing campaign is going to cost. While they may be happy – even excited – about the results of marketing, they are often turned off by the perceived expense.

This situation accounts for one of the major barriers to marketing in the minds of healthcare executives. While for-profit organizations such as pharmaceutical companies see marketing expenses as a normal cost of doing business, hospitals and physicians with limited experience in this regard are often unprepared for the marketing price tag. In a cost-conscious environment, healthcare executives have concerns over the expense involved in implementing a marketing campaign, not to mention the resources required for establishing a formal marketing program.

There are generally two viable responses to healthcare executives who suffer from the "sticker shock" that often accompanies a marketing initiative. The first is the standard admonition: You get what you pay for. It is always possible to cut corners but with most marketing campaigns you only have one opportunity to get it right. There is only going to be *one* grand opening for the new hospital wing, *one* introduction of the new service, and *one* introduction of the organization's new brand.

These are activities for which it may be difficult to quantify the benefits of doing it right, but there can certainly be significant fallout from doing it wrong.

The second response is that marketing doesn't *have* to cost a lot. Indeed, much of the marketing that the organization is already doing is relatively low cost, and even more formal marketing efforts can often be done inexpensively. Most marketing involves little or no cost – at least in terms of out-of-pocket expenses – and an amazing amount of marketing can be built into routine corporate activities.

Marketing as an Investment

Administrators have a tendency to perceive of marketing as a necessary evil, a cost center that cannot be avoided in today's healthcare environment. This commonly held negative view reflects a misunderstanding of marketing and creates an artificial impediment to incorporating marketing into the organization. A more positive stance views marketing as an investment that, if properly made, will pay dividends not only today but also in the future. (Of course, this assumes the ability to measure the return on marketing investment, but more about that later.)

Marketing expenditures should not be made only for short-term gains, but as an investment intended to reap future benefits. At one time in healthcare the bulk of marketing was geared toward "making the sale," getting that customer in the door, or signing them up for an affinity program. Too much attention was paid to getting a $500 sale rather than obtaining a customer for life who would ultimately spend $250,000 on healthcare. The *real* goal of marketing should be to establish a relationship that will pay long-term dividends.

A useful example of marketing as relationship development is the patient satisfaction survey conducted after discharge. Ostensibly, the intent of the survey is to measure customer satisfaction for purposes of improving service in the future. But the simple process of collecting satisfaction data can be viewed as an opportunity for developing a relationship with the patient and the patient's family. Seeking input from customers and otherwise engaging them in dialog can serve multiple purposes. Seen in this light, the $15 that seems high for a completed satisfaction questionnaire doesn't look like much of an investment for solidifying a relationship with a potential lifelong customer.

On the topic of the long-term impact of marketing, don't forget the contribution that marketing makes to the strategic direction of the organization. How much is it worth to the organization to be able to identify a strategy that will result in increased productivity and profitability over time? The investment in the marketing research component by itself should pay handsome benefits to the organization by virtue of the guidance marketing provides in positioning the organization within the marketplace.

Rethinking Marketing Costs

Ideally, marketing expenses should be thought of as an investment in future productivity and future profitability. And like all *investments* they share a certain amount of risk, a certain amount of faith, and a certain amount of trust among participants. Risk because the marketplace is constantly changing and shifting its priorities very much like the stock market does. Faith because there are fundamental rules that can be counted on to assure the marketing efforts serve to generate an acceptable return on investment. Trust because good marketing is a team endeavor, a joint venture, and a collaboration among people with a common goal. Whether to spend a little or a lot is not the real question. The real question is: What do you ultimately want to accomplish? Answer this basic question and the issue of expensive high-end marketing versus marketing-on-the-cheap will be essentially answered.

A more progressive stance views marketing as an investment that if properly made will pay huge dividends not only today but in the future. Marketing efforts that are invested in effective advertisements, attracting quality medical or nursing staff, solidifying relationships with referral agents, generating donations or raising awareness of a new service can pay immediate dividends and provide long-term benefits.

Marketing Expenditures in Healthcare

In examining the costs involved in marketing, it is important to consider the full range of activities subsumed under the marketing umbrella. While advertising costs are likely to stand out in the budget, they really account for only a fraction of total marketing expenditures. Once consideration is given to salaries, research expenses, administrative costs, etc., the importance of advertising expenditures diminishes. Indeed, as seen in the data provided by the Society for Healthcare Strategy and Market Development shown in Box 7.1, advertising expenditures account for about one-third of marketing costs for hospitals – typically the biggest spenders among healthcare organizations. The distribution of marketing expenditures shown in Box 7.1 reflects the range of marketing activities characterizing large healthcare organizations.

Marketing expenses should never be determined in a vacuum. That is, they should be planned within the operating limitations of the overall budget. They also have to take into account that some markets are far more expensive to operate in than others. Some marketing activities are more expensive than others, some competitors are far bigger than others, and some types of health services are more expensive to promote than others.

There are, in fact, decisions that can be made throughout the marketing planning process to match tactical expenses to strategic priorities and keep them in line with the overall budget. Marketing expenses represent an investment in the future, and the true benefits of a marketing effort may only be apparent some time after the campaign is completed.

Box 7.1 Comparative marketing expense statistics

The Society for Healthcare Strategy and Market Development has released figures for 2004 on marketing expenditures by a sample of 273 hospitals nationwide. These figures are restricted to hospital expenditures and reflect actual practice rather than any ideal allocation of resources. Nevertheless, they provide a framework within which to view the marketing expenditures for any healthcare organization.

Average marketing/communication budget	$1,010,000
Percent of net hospital revenue	0.56%

Allocation by marketing function:

Salaries	25%
Advertising	36%
Publications	10%
Collateral materials	8%
Community events/giveaways	8%
Marketing research	3%
Website management	3%
Call center expenses	2%
Other expenses	7%

Allocation of advertising expenses:

Newspapers/magazines	35%
Television	16%
Radio	14%
Yellow pages	10%
Direct mail	10%
Outdoor	9%
Internet	2%
Other	4%

Source: Society for Healthcare Strategy and Market Development (2005).

Paying for Marketing Expertise

At some point, every organization faces the question of whether to create marketing expertise inside the organization or use the services of an outside advertising or public relations firm. Any significant marketing initiative is likely to require expertise not available within the organization. The effort may be as simple as coming up with a name for a new service or as complex as the development of a branding campaign. Marketing professionals know how to do these things and know how to do them right. These are skills that are not likely to be found within the typical healthcare organization.

The idea is to get the best talent the budget can support, so there is no hard and fast rule about whether it is better to make or buy. In general, the same pros and cons exist as with the make-or-buy debate related to marketing research. Outside marketing consultants tend to have broad experience, expertise specific to the challenge at hand, and that all-important objective outside perspective. Using in-house resources may appear to be less expensive, but if internal staff do not have the skills, what they cost is irrelevant. In putting together a marketing team, the trick, of course, is to acquire the best talent available in order to increase the likelihood of success. The right marketing manager, just like a coach, can mix up his team and put experience where it is needed most.

There is one other variable here that is also important. In marketing *Time is Money*. If you have a huge budget you can build awareness very fast. You can literally buy a lot of time and space. If you have a small budget it will take longer to move the needle. For example, advertising is more expensive but has the potential for immediate impact. Public relations is much less expensive but usually much slower to show results. The trick is to develop a mix of activities that allows the marketing problem to be attacked from a variety of angles.

It is important to not be turned off by what might be perceived as a high hourly fee for marketing consultation and creative services. You are not just buying an hour's labor, you're buying the experience and expertise that's behind that hour – and this could be considered priceless. If you have engaged the right marketing professional, that person is going to give you much more than an hour's work and may provide insights into the next marketing opportunity. (Box 7.2 presents data on the use of outside resources by the nation's hospitals.)

Box 7.2 Use of outside agencies

The Society for Healthcare Strategy and Market Development has released figures for 2004 on marketing activities for a sample of 273 hospitals nationwide. These figures provide a framework within which to view the outsourcing of marketing activities for any healthcare organization.

Activity	Percent Using Outside Agencies
Patient satisfaction tracking	81%
Collateral materials	77%
Advertising	76%
Marketing research	64%
Internet strategy/web development	50%
Strategic planning	34%
Marketing consulting	31%
Public relations	20%
Physician strategy development	18%
Event planning	17%

Source: Society for Healthcare Strategy and Market Development (2005).

Investing in Marketing Resources

The costs involved in the establishment of a marketing department are generally the same as for the creation of any other department. The components to be considered should support marketing research, marketing planning, marketing implementation, and marketing management. These could be represented by one person and some support staff, a team of marketing professionals, or some combination of internal and external resources. The dollars budgeted should include both the direct and indirect costs involved.

Core personnel costs (salary and benefits) should be considered along with any recruiting and training costs. Standard overhead costs associated with operating the department and supporting the staff should be considered. Telecommunication and IT costs must be factored in, as well as travel expenses and professional development costs (e.g., dues and subscriptions).

The costs associated with marketing research must also be factored into the equation, including both ongoing infrastructure expenses and nonrecurring expenses. These costs would include, in addition to the salaries of research personnel, the costs associated with data acquisition and management, any out-of-pocket research expenses (e.g., for telephone surveys and market analyses), and any evaluation costs above and beyond core staffing.

Presumably, the marketing department will be involved in the development of collateral materials (e.g., letterhead, business cards, and brochures), and the costs associated with the design and production of these materials should be factored into the budget. Expenses involved in trade show exhibits and other sales-oriented events, along with any expenses associated with promotional items (e.g., key chains, pens, or refrigerator magnets) should also be considered.

Careful consideration should be given to the production of collateral materials. This is one area where executives may think with their egos rather than their marketing sense. Full-color brochures may be attractive and contribute in some way to the furtherance of organizational goals but, given that they are likely to be distributed to employees or existing customers, they may constitute "preaching to the choir." They also may drain resources away from other marketing activities while failing to generate any new business. (In view of the cost of collateral materials, a surge in "e-collateral" among healthcare providers is in evidence. This approach reduces the need for expensive print collateral while accommodating the preferences of consumers for easily accessed, customized materials.)

With regard to a specific marketing campaign, budget items should address the cost for creative work, outside agency expenses, production costs for marketing materials, and direct mail expenses. Of course, a big ticket item is likely to be media expenses. Television, radio, and newspaper advertising expenses often approximate the cost of operating the department.

An important consideration throughout this process is the nonmonetary investment in marketing. This investment includes the cost of intangibles that do not show up on the bottom line. At the top of this list should be the time and energy committed on the part of senior management are drawn away from other tasks.

Other indirect costs include the time and opportunity costs of employees who may be required to spend time with the marketing staff as they develop the concept. Resources are likely to be required from the research, planning, or business development staff, as well as input from IT and medical records staff. Marketing input is typically not written into the job description for such positions, and time will have to be carved out from other activities. This is an important consideration in establishing an in-house marketing capability. (Table 7.1 presents a sample marketing budget template.)

Getting the Most Bang for the Buck

A key to squeezing the most benefit out of marketing efforts is to assure that all such efforts serve multiple purposes. This is perhaps most difficult to achieve with advertising which, by definite, has a very specific purpose. Even here, a print or electronic advertisement for a new service should, at the same time, contribute to an enhanced image of the organization. Realistically, most consumers viewing the ad are not going to be immediate customers for the new service. But at some point they are likely to be customers for *some* hospital service. If the image that was conveyed is first class, the consumer is likely to remember this years from now.

As has been pointed out elsewhere (Thomas and Calhoun, 2007), much of what falls under the heading of marketing does not have to be costly. There are a number of activities supportive of marketing that can be carried out, some of them inherent aspects of the operation that involve little or no out-of-pocket expenditures. There are other promotional techniques that are both inexpensive and effective.

The typical healthcare organization carries out many activities without any thought to their marketing significance. These include such diverse activities as utilizing a state-of-the-art practice management system, establishing efficient admission and discharge procedures, generating bills that are easily understood, providing insurance submission guidance, and even maintaining an attractive and therapeutic physical plant. Although health professionals are becoming increasingly aware of the potential implications of functions that appear to be far removed from patient care, these activities are typically not carried out with marketing in mind. The trick is to tweak functions that are already being performed in order to turn them into marketing assets.

There are some activities that constitute marketing that might not be obvious. These include such activities as communicating developments and new services to employees, providing a newsletter to patients and other customers, sponsoring a series of patient education programs, following up with patients after discharge, facilitating e-mail contact with providers, providing timely and thoughtful feedback to referring physicians, and conducting patient satisfaction surveys, among many other activities. These are typically routine activities generally considered part of "the cost of doing business" but *not* considered from a marketing perspective.

There are a number of activities that are more directly considered under the marketing umbrella that can be carried out inexpensively (and more about this in a later chapter). Many public relations activities cost virtually nothing beyond the

Table 7.1 Sample marketing budget template.

Marketing expenditures	Quarter I Dollars %	Quarter II Dollars %	Quarter III Dollars %	Quarter IV Dollars %
Advertising				
Newspaper				
Magazines				
Trade publications				
Radio				
Outdoor				
Television				
Specialty items				
Direct Mail				
Point of purchase				
Co-op ads				
Production/creative				
Sales promotion				
Brochures/flyers				
Trade shows				
Newsletters				
Customer services				
Decor/display				
Community events				
Clerical				
Managerial				
Secretarial				
Telephone				
Travel				
Postage				
Supplies				
Sales force expenditures				
Motivation program				
Recruiting				
Salaries and benefits				
Telephone				
Training program				
Travel				
Professional membership				
Subscriptions				
Marketing research				
Computer time				
Salaries and benefits				
Supplies				
Telephone				
Travel				
Miscellaneous				
Total budget				

staff effort that is already being paid for. News items and articles in publications constitute free advertising and often require minimal effort. Visible participation by staff in community activities and the sponsorship of community events are low-cost activities that often generate considerable return. Public service announcements available to not-for-profit organizations involve only the cost of laying out the ad and can generate considerable response. Activities of the communication staff should all be considered marketing efforts. In-house publications should be the prime vehicle for internal marketing, and newsletters distributed to patients and potential patients should communicate useful information and lay the groundwork for future service utilization.

Even if paid advertising is unavoidable, there are low-cost options here that should be considered. Banner ads run in newspapers and links on related web sites are inexpensive and can generate significant exposure. Listings in the appropriate directories (usually free) can also be a source of referrals. Any opportunity for co-marketing should be taken advantage of. (Box 7.3 presents data on comparative media advertising costs.)

Box 7.3 Comparative advertising costs

The figures provided below provide current examples of the advertising costs for various media. The actual cost will depend on such factors as the size, duration and timing of the advertisement. Costs can be expected to vary widely from market to market. These figures should be used only as a comparative rule-of-thumb.

Newspapers – $1,300 per week for 2″ × 2″ ad

Television – $200,000 for one 30-second commercial (during prime-time)

Direct Mail – $1,500 for 1,000 4 × 6 postcards (including postage)

Radio – $90–$120 per week on a rotator (prices higher if time slots for ad are selective)

Magazines – $1,200–$5,000 per month or per issue (depends on ad size and demographics)

Outdoor (billboard) – $3,000 to do artwork and install media on billboard; rates depend on impress level, ranges from $5,000 to $500,000 (the higher the qualify of the artwork and the larger the demographic group, the higher the price); minimum contract is 16 weeks

Online – $0.60 pay-per-click or $1,200–$1,800 a month for aggressive campaigns (does not include search engine optimization) or $200–$1,200 per year per banner ad on websites

Source: Inland Empire Small Business Development Center. Downloaded from http://www.iesbdc.org/resources/Major%20Media%20Types.doc 3/15/07.

Reference

Thomas, Richard K., and Michael Calhoun (2007). *Marketing Matters: A Guide for Healthcare Executives*. Chicago: Health Administration Press.

Chapter 8
Market Positioning and Strategy Development

The natural tendency to rush into a marketing initiative must be tempered by the need to consider the organization's position in the market and formulate an appropriate strategy. A well thought out marketing strategy provides guidelines for the development of the marketing initiative and allows for thoughtful selection from the various marketing techniques that are available. This chapter emphasizes the importance of developing a position for your organization within its market and developing a strategy that reinforces that position.

Positioning the Organization

An appreciation of two concepts – positioning and strategy development – are essential for effective marketing. "Positioning" refers to the way a product or organization is perceived by the target audience relative to other products or organizations. The position a healthcare organization occupies within the pecking order of the marketplace reflects the manner in which it is known within the community.

There are, in fact, *two* positions that an organization can occupy – one determined by statistics and the other by perceptions. On the one hand, there are statistical indicators of its position such as market share, penetration rates, service line dominance and so forth that offer an objective picture. On the other, there is the position that exists in the public's mind or the subjective position. Marketing should function to enhance the organization's objective position while assuring a favorable perception on the subjective dimension.

As with other attributes discussed previously, each organization should establish its own position in the market and not let someone else dictate it. This position should reflect how it wants to be known in the market. If the staff of the organization does not proactively establish and manage its position, the marketplace will establish one. A major objective of marketing, then, should be to maintain control over the organization's position.

It is important to understand the characteristics of the market for both positioning and strategy development purposes. This means knowing the characteristics of the target audience and the competition. The market should be assessed in terms of its demographic characteristics, health status and utilization patterns. This should also involve an assessment of the competitive situation. Since an understanding of the competition is necessary for the development of an effective positioning strategy.

Determining the organization's objective position in the market requires access to both internal and external data and, ultimately, the ability to interface the two. While an experienced researcher can analyze the positions of competitors and measure how strong these positions are, grassroots research may be required to determine the subjective dimension of the organization's position. This might involve consumer surveys (including patient satisfaction research), focus groups and/or in-depth interviews with community leaders, health professionals, policy makers and the organization's employees. (Box 8.1 discusses issues to take into consideration when positioning the organization.)

Positioning can occur at different levels within the organization, especially in the case of a large health system. While the positioning of all components of the organization should generally align, there may be reasons to position different subdivisions, service lines or products in different ways. Similarly, differential positioning may be in place for different aspects of the marketing mix. Thus, one of the four Ps – product, price, place and promotion – may be emphasized over the other three, or different services may be associated with different marketing positions. For example, fixed inpatient services may be positioned in terms of the product while the network of urgent care centers is positioned in terms of place.

Box 8.1 Positioning considerations

The one thing that might be worse than not having a position is the establishment of an indefensible position. An inappropriately positioned organization (or service or facility) will not contribute to organizational success no matter what resources are invested. Staking out an inappropriate positon becomes more of a liability than an asset. Ultimately, the position chosen should be related to the organization's mission, be unique, be credible, and easily remembered.

Questions that might be asked in assessing the organization's position include:

- What is the market share currently controlled by the organization or the particular service?
- How has this market share changed over time?
- What unique attributes can the organization or service claim?
- How is the organization or service perceived relative to its competitors?
- Do consumers see the organization or service as it sees itself?
- How do other providers perceive the organization or service?

Determining Your Position

As noted above, there are two dimensions along which an organization or product might be assessed – an objective one and a subjective one. An objective determination of market share requires information on the market and the players that occupy that space. In order to calculate market share, it is necessary to identify the organization's competitors, profile them and determine their level of activity. This will typically require data on patient visits, hospital admissions, revenue and any other indicator that will contribute to an understanding of the relative position of the various players in the marketplace.

The first step, of course, is acquiring data on your organization. Depending on the market share indicator being considered, this will mean compiling data on patient volumes, revenue, and relevant utilization patterns. This may also require decomposing the data into meaningful components. For example, if the hospital wants to determine its OB market share, figures on overall admissions are not very helpful. Data need to be acquired on OB-specific admissions, procedures, etc., to allow for an apples-to-apples comparison. Similarly, if the Medicare population is being targeted, data on the admissions of commercially insured patients are not very relevant. Here, as elsewhere, data acquisition should match the need.

Most organizations are going to have internal data that provides the basis for self-assessment. Obtaining the necessary market intelligence for profiling competitors may be more of a challenge. In some markets there may be data repositories that are maintained that can be assessed to determine the activity of various competitors. At the very least, it may be possible to determine the aggregate amount of activity (e.g., admissions, procedures) in order to determine *your* market share. (Box 8.2 presents an example of a competitor "spec sheet.")

Box 8.2 Competitor spec sheet

Accurately determining an organization's market share requires information on the competitors that exist in the marketplace. The more that is known about them, the easier it will be to assess the organization's position in the market. To this end, it might be worthwhile to develop a "spec sheet" that profiles competitors in terms of relevant characteristics. Such a sheet might be set up as follows:

Competitor Organization	Estimated Patient Volume	Perceived Market Share	Perceived Strengths	Relevant Weaknesses	Trends
1.					
2.					
3.					
4.					
5.					

In situations where there is very little data available it may be necessary to synthetically generate utilization figures using computer models. The analyst needs access to population estimates and projections and access to relevant utilization rates in order to do this. Using this methodology it is possible to model utilization levels for the service in question and then determine your organization's share of the total. (For those who do not want to go to this trouble, there are consultants that can calculate these figures.)

Determining the subjective perception of your organization or service requires a different approach. Unless your organization regularly collects information on consumer perceptions or some other organization does this for the market area, it will probably be necessary to conduct a consumer survey. If you are already conducting patient satisfaction surveys, it may be possible to obtain some information through this means on the relative perceptions of your organization and its competition. However, your patients may have had limited exposure to other providers or services and thus be unable to provide much information.

Ultimately, it may be necessary to conduct a survey of consumers in the community. The methodology used, the size of the sample and the form the questions take all require a certain level of expertise. If this expertise is not available in-house, it may be necessary to engage consultant to assist in this process. (Chapter 4 on market research may be helpful in planning a consumer survey.)

Taking the pulse of the market is a challenge, and careful attention has to be paid to the wording of the questions being asked. The intent is to determine perceptions of your organization or a specific service relative to that of competitors. Care has to be taken to assure that the responses are not biased in one way or another. Again, a research consultant may be useful in this regard. There is also the option of piggy-backing data collection onto an existing survey that is being conducted. In many markets, there are organizations that regularly conduct consumer surveys and some, in fact, may already be conducting surveys on health-related issues. It is often more cost-effective to leverage an existing survey than to develop your own.

Strategy Development

The term "strategy" is used in a variety of ways but, for our purposes, it refers to the generalized approach that is taken in meeting the challenges of the market. The strategy sets the tone for any marketing activities (tactics) and establishes the parameters within which the marketer must operate. The strategy that is chosen will determine the characteristics of the marketing plan and inform any subsequent marketing initiatives. (Box 8.3 provides the reasons why strategy development is important.)

In today's environment, few healthcare organizations can successfully compete without a well thought out strategy. Strategies serve numerous purposes for the organization, and there are a number of different strategies that might be employed. Various strategic options must be assessed and the relevance of the traditional four

> **Box 8.3** Why establish a strategy?
> - Provide direction for the organization or program.
> - Focus the effort on one of many possible options.
> - Unify the organization's actions.
> - Differentiate the organization.
> - Customize the organization's promotions.
> - Guide allocation of marketing resources.
> - Support decision making within the organization.
> - Provide a competitive edge for the organization.

Ps of marketing – product, price, place and promotion – for strategy development considered.

Marketers often think in terms of different "levels" at which strategies might be developed. These could include a "corporate strategy" that deals with the overall development of an organization's business activities, a "business strategy" that indicates how to approach a particular product and/or market, or a "marketing strategy" focusing on one or more aspects of the marketing mix. The marketing strategy is the most relevant for our purposes and might be thought of as the logic through which an organization hopes to achieve its marketing objectives.

Ideally strategies are carefully thought out and deliberately formulated as a result of strategic planning. However, the lack of an articulated strategy does not mean that no strategy exists. Acts of commission or omission ultimately serve to create a strategy. Indeed, the lack of a strategy could technically be considered a strategic approach, and many healthcare organizations end up with *de facto* strategies that were not deliberately formulated. In effect, this approachets the market (or even the competition) set your strategy.

The rational choices that must be made in healthcare require a context that establishes the goals and objectives to be met, as well as agreed-upon criteria for decision making. It is the organization's strategic plan treat provides the framework within which to establish goals and objectives and make marketing decisions.

Strategic Options

A number of factors must be considered in the selection of a strategy. Marketers must consider the nature of the organization and its mission, the characteristics of the market (and, more specifically, the organization's customers), and the nature of the competition. Ultimately, the strategy chosen will determine how the "public" perceives the organization. Ideally, the strategy employed for any marketing initiative will support the organization's mission statement and reflect the

Box 8.4 The SWOT analysis

The SWOT analysis has become an increasingly common technique for assessing the position of a healthcare organization within its market. The SWOT analysis involves an examination of the organization, its environment, and the manner in which the organization and its environment interact. This is an important tool for strategists and marketers and one that has numerous applications in healthcare. The SWOT analysis can be done for departments within organizations as well as total organizations. Factors within both the broader social environment and narrower competitive environment should be considered.

The SWOT analysis involves an examination of the *strengths, weaknesses, opportunities* and *threats* relative to an organization or a product. A strength can be thought of as a particular skill or distinctive competence, which the organization possesses and which will aid it in achieving its stated objectives. These would include marketing capabilities, management skills, the organization's image, financial resources and any number of other assets. A weakness refers to any aspect of the organization that might undermine the achievement of specific objectives. These might include inadequate working capital, poor management skills, a lack of certain services, personnel shortages and any of a variety of other weaknesses.

An opportunity is any feature of the internal or external environment that creates conditions which are advantageous to the organization in relation to its goals and objectives. Opportunities may take a variety of forms, such as gaps in the market, new sources of reimbursement, demographic changes, weaknesses among competitors, and so forth. A threat is any environmental development that hinders the achievement of organizational objectives. Threats may come in the form of competitive activity, unfavorable demographic trends, unanticipated reimbursement changes, etc.

The SWOT analysis should include input from any quantitative research that is being conducted as well as from the interviews that are administered. Because the strengths, weaknesses, opportunities and threats that are identified will guide further development of the plan, it is important that consensus be reached on these attributes before proceeding with the planning process.

strategy embodied in the organization's strategic plan. Thus, if the organization's strategy involves positioning itself as a "caring" organization, the organization's marketing initiatives should support this approach.

Unfortunately, there is not a standard list of strategies from which the organization can choose. Each situation is likely to be unique and call for creativity in strategy selection. One of the analytical approaches that can be pursued in determining the appropriate strategy is the SWOT analysis. The SWOT analysis examines the strengths, weaknesses, opportunities, and threats for a particular market, organization, or product. The SWOT analysis should provide a basis for subsequent strategy development, since it simultaneously considers several dimensions of the situation.

The assessment of the strengths of the organization will indicate the attributes on which the strategist should capitalize. The weaknesses indicate organizational deficiencies that should be minimized or ameliorated. The threats indicate potentially harmful aspects of the organization or environment that should be neutralized by means of the strategic thrust. Of the four dimensions, opportunities have perhaps the most salience for strategy development, since an implicit goal of the strategy chosen should be to exploit opportunities that exist in the marketplace. (The SWOT analysis is discussed further in Box 8.4.)

A number of approaches can be taken to strategy development. The approach can focus on the market and, thus, concentrate on market-oriented strategies. It can focus on a product or a service line and involve a product-oriented strategy. The approach can address an aspect of the marketing mix, as in the case of a pricing strategy, or it can cut across the marketing mix and be broader in its scope.

One approach to strategy selection might be based on the product/market mix. For example, a *market penetration strategy* (existing market/existing product) would involve efforts to extract more sales and greater usage out of existing customers, acquire customers from competitors; and/or convert nonusers into users. A *market development strategy* (new market/existing product) would involve the identification of new market sectors based on different benefit profiles, establishing new distribution channels, identifying new marketing approaches, and identifying underserved geographic areas.

A *new product or service development strategy* (existing market/new product) would call for modifications of existing services, introducing differing quality levels and/or developing entirely new products. A *diversification strategy* (new market/new product) would involve actions such as horizontal and/or vertical integration, concentric diversification, and conglomerate diversification. (Box 8.5 presents some examples of strategic approaches and criteria for their use.)

Box 8.5 Strategy options and criteria for their use

A number of examples of market-oriented strategies utilized in healthcare can be identified. Examples of these include:

- *Dominance strategy* whereby the number one player in the market opts to focus on maintaining this position.
- *Second fiddle strategy* in which the "runner-up" in the market concedes its second-fiddle status and acts accordingly, adopting what might also be called a "market follower" strategy.
- *Frontal attack strategy* in which the organization decides to confront the market leader or major competitors head on.
- *Niche strategy* in which the organization concedes it cannot successfully compete for the mainstream market but instead concentrates on niche markets based on geography, population groups, or selected services.
- *Flanking strategy* in which the organization "outflanks" the competition by entering new markets, cultivating new populations, or offering fringe products.

Strategy and the Four Ps

One approach to selecting a strategy reflects the role of the marketing mix in setting the strategic direction. The strategy could focus on any dimension of the four Ps or reflect a strategy that cuts across two or more of them.

Product Strategies

Product strategies focus on a good or service offered by the organization. The strategy is built around the qualities of the product, and the marketing approach attempts to capitalize on this. A product-oriented approach might focus on a *unique selling proposition* and relate to the ability of the organization to establish and communicate a distinct product benefit which competitors cannot match.

A *positioning strategy* attempts to define in the consumer's mind the comparisons between one product and another. The task is to identify weaknesses in competing products and strengths in your own which can be reinforced so as to gain a competitive edge. Positioning indicates to customers how the company differs from current or potential competitors. Positioning strategies can focus on different aspects of the products and the position could be established with regard to product features, benefits, usage, or users.

Pricing Strategies

Healthcare providers have seldom employed pricing strategies in the past. End-users of health services usually do not know the prices of the services they consume, and the primary decision maker with regard to the purchase of services, the physician, seldom takes pricing into consideration. Further, the amount of reimbursement for services from third-party payers was often established independently of the price set by the provider. For these reasons, healthcare has provided few opportunities for patient care organizations to compete in terms of price. On the other hand, more "retail" oriented healthcare businesses such as personal health product manufacturers are likely to employ pricing strategies in much the same manner as other producers of other consumer goods.

Despite these barriers to the use of pricing strategies, there are growing numbers of providers that are competing on price. These primarily reflect the growing importance of elective procedures in the industry. Price can be used as a basis for competition for services that are discretionary and typically paid for out of pocket. Most cosmetic surgery would fall into this category and, as competition has increased among ophthalmic surgeons, ophthalmologists performing laser eye surgery have begun to compete on the basis of price.

Place Strategies

Place focuses on the manner of distribution for a good or service, and in healthcare this typically refers to the place where services are rendered. An important aspect of "place" is the channel of distribution, or the path a good or service takes as it travels from the producer to the consumer.

A variety of channel(s) of distribution are used to deliver health services. Primary care centers are typically located near potential patients (e.g., in neighborhoods and/or heavily populated residential areas) while tertiary services are concentrated in medical centers, regardless of the proximity to population centers. Emergency services represent a combination of distribution methods, since the ambulances travel to the patient but then take the patient to the hospital for treatment.

Historically, little emphasis was placed on the location of service outlets in healthcare. The bulk of the care was provided by hospitals, and patients were expected to travel to wherever the hospital was located. The same attitude was evinced on the part of physicians (especially specialists). As the focus of healthcare has shifted away from the inpatient setting to the outpatient setting, healthcare providers have been forced to pay attention to the location of services.

This new emphasis on place has also been encouraged by the employers and business coalitions that pay a large share of the healthcare bill. Employers want their employees to have convenient access to services, not only to assure patient satisfaction but to limit the time lost from work due to the use of occupational health services. Health maintenance organizations and other health plans seek to establish networks of providers that are distributed in a manner that meets the needs of their enrollee populations. The contemporary consumer demands convenient locations and, in cases where locations cannot be changed, healthcare providers are attempting to enhance effective access through more efficient patient processing methods and more appealing facilities.

Promotional Strategies

The most visible type of strategy employed by healthcare organizations is likely to be one that relates to the promotion of the organization or its services. Much of the marketing effort on the part of healthcare providers over the past two decades has focused on advertising, direct mail and other promotional strategies. The limitations on competition based on product, price and place have encouraged healthcare providers to attempt to differentiate themselves through promotional strategies.

The promotional strategy should reflect the approach to the market that the organization has chosen. If the organization has adopted an aggressive, hard-sell approach to the market, the promotional strategy should reflect this. Conversely, the organization may have adopted a soft-sell approach, and this would be reflected in initiatives meant to educate the market.

A promotions-oriented strategy can take a variety of forms. For example, a *resonance strategy* is one which "strikes a chord" with the consumer. The intention is to portray a lifestyle orientation which is synonymous with the target group and one which is easily recognizable. Such an approach might be advocated for the promotion of a hospital-based fitness center. An *emotional strategy* may be adopted by healthcare organizations wishing to play on, as well as play to, the emotions of the consumer, as in the case of children's health services. (Box 8.6 describes the use of branding as a strategy.)

Box 8.6 Branding as a strategy

A "brand" is a name, term, symbol, or design (or combination thereof) intended to characterize the goods or services of an organization and to differentiate it from its competitors. An effective brand name evokes positive associations with the organization. The brand image indicates what business the company is in, what benefit it provides, and why it is better than the competition. Brand associations are the attributes that consumers think of when they hear or see the brand name. Therefore, the logic behind branding is simple: if consumers are more familiar with a company's brand, they are more likely to purchase the company's products.

The following critical success factors must be considered when developing and implementing a branding strategy:

- Make sure that the organization or service is amenable to branding. Not everything is.
- Make sure the brand can be linked back to the organization's mission statement and business model.
- Carefully think through the implications of creating a brand (including the unintended consequences).
- Envision the proposed brand from the perspective of the target audience.
- Promote the brand internally before rolling it out in the marketplace.
- Don't use branding to try to overcome an inferior product or poor service.
- Make sure that the necessary data for tracking the impact of the branding strategy will be available.
- Continuously update and revitalize the brand.

Regardless of the approach taken to strategy development, there are certain guidelines that should be followed. Box 8.7 offers a checklist that could be used in strategy selection.

Box 8.7 Strategy development checklist

In developing a strategy for the marketing of an organization (or idea or service) a number of factors must be taken into consideration. While the questions presented below do not represent an exhaustive list, they do indicate the types of issues that should be raised.

- What is the organization's mission statement and what are the implications of this statement for strategy formulation?
- What are the strengths and weaknesses of the organization (or idea or service) that is to be marketed?
- What niche in the marketplace (e.g., type of service, target population, or geographic area) is this strategy meant to address?
- How is the organization or service positioned in the market and what are the implications of this positioning for strategy formulation?
- Does the organization or service have a unique selling proposition that can be built on?
- How is the competition positioned in the market and what are the implications of this for strategy development?
- What aspect(s) of the marketing mix (e.g., product, price, place, promotion) has the most saliency with regard to strategy formulation?
- What barriers exist in the market that may deter the use of a particular strategy?
- What are the unintended consequences that might result from the implementation of a particular strategy?

Chapter 9
Choosing Among Promotional Options

For most people, the rubber hits the road in marketing when various promotional techniques are implemented. Marketing techniques such as advertising, public relations and other types of promotions are the tools of the marketing practitioner, and, whether you are involved in hands-on marketing activities or have oversight for your organization's marketing efforts, it's important to know the ends-and-outs of promotional techniques. This chapter provides an overview of the "standard" promotional techniques that are used by healthcare marketers.

Promotion: The Business End of Marketing

Promotion is the action component of the marketing mix. "Promotion" refers to any of the variety of techniques used to reach customers and potential customers with the purpose of promoting an idea, organization, or product. The range of "traditional" promotional activities includes such familiar techniques as public relations, advertising, sales, and direct marketing, as well as other less familiar forms of promotion. The "promotional mix" refers to the combination of these elements that constitutes the chosen promotional strategy.

The choice of promotional technique will reflect a number of factors and the nature of the *organization* is a key factor determining the promotional approach. A large, multi-unit organization is likely to take a different approach than a small, family-run operation, with the differential availability of resources likely to be a consideration. Not-for-profits are likely to take a different approach from for-profit healthcare organizations. Organizations involved in direct patient care are likely to take a different approach from those that provide support services.

The choice of promotional approach will also be influenced by the nature of the *product* being offered. The promotion of consumer health products calls for a different approach than the promotion of personal health services. Episodic care calls for a different approach than care based on long-term relationships. Elective services are amenable to different types of approaches than nonelective services.

The characteristics of the *community* also play a role in the choice of promotional approach. The "culture" of the community may render some approaches more acceptable than others, and the local climate may limit the use of some approaches. An in-your-face approach to the promotion of certain products may generate a negative backlash in some communities. Different media options may be more or less available in a particular market.

The nature of the *target audience* will also be a factor in the choice of promotional approach. Target audiences with different demographic or psychographic characteristics call for different promotional techniques. The size and geographic distribution of the audience, along with lifestyle orientation, may be factors. Different segments of the population are responsive to different media, and such factors as consumer access to cable television or the Internet may come into play.

Standard Promotional Techniques

Each promotional technique has certain traits that influence its applicability to a certain situation. The criteria discussed above must be matched with the characteristics of the various promotional techniques to assure the compatibility of the task and the tool. Each of these techniques is described below.

Public Relations and Communication

Public relations (PR) make uses of publicity and other non-paid forms of promotion and information dissemination to influence feelings, opinions or beliefs about an organization and its services. Core functions include announcements to the media and the distribution of news releases describing some newsworthy event or activity.

Public relations include:

- Collateral materials (including e-collateral)
  - Brochures
  - Letterhead
  - Business cards
- Press releases
- Press conferences
- Distribution of feature stories to the media
- Public service announcements
- Event sponsorships

Various other forms of communication might also be considered under the publicity heading. Healthcare organizations typically establish mechanisms for communicating with their various publics (both internal and external). Communication staff develops materials for dissemination to the public and the employees of the organization. Examples of these include internal newsletters, publications geared to relevant customers groups (e.g., patients, enrollees), and patient education materials. Separate communication departments may be established, or this function may overlap with the public relations or community outreach functions.

The public service announcement (PSA) uses advertising as a vehicle for publicity. The PSA is an advertisement or commercial that is carried by a medium at no cost as a public service to its readers, viewers, or listeners. This could be carried on radio or television or be printed in newspaper or magazine. Billboards are also used for public service announcements. While the no-cost aspect is appealing, the downside is that the advertising organization has no control over the placement or timing of PSA presentation. Further, many media are no longer required to provide free space/time for public service announcements.

Another form of publicity involves sponsorships on the part of the organization – corporate financial backing for a project or event in return for public exposure and goodwill. The sponsor typically does not run an advertisement but may be mentioned in terms of "brought to you by." A sponsorship provides the sponsor with potentially substantial media coverage and may contribute to improved employee morale.

Publicity might also be generated by means of a campaign spokesperson. These could be athletes, entertainers, community leaders or others who are thought to influence the public mindset. They could also be animated characters that are known to the public or characters created specifically for this promotion. By associating the organization with a recognizable person or character, the campaign benefits from the goodwill generated by the spokesperson.

Community Outreach

Community outreach is a form of marketing that seeks to present the programs of the organization to the community and establish relationships with community organizations. Community outreach may involve episodic activities such as health fairs and educational programs for community residents. This function may also include on-going initiatives involving outreach workers who are visible within the community on a recurring basis. While the benefits of community outreach activities are not as easily measured as some more direct marketing activities, the organization often gains customers as a result of its health screening activities, follow-up from educational seminars, or outreach worker referrals.

Networking

Networking involves developing and nurturing relationships with individuals and organizations with which mutually beneficial transactions might be carried out. As such, networking is probably the least formal of the various promotional techniques used in healthcare. Physicians and other clinicians, who until recently would never have considering advertising, actively network among their colleagues. Such networking might take place at sporting events, social affairs or at the country club. Networking is particularly effective when dealing with parties with whom it is particularly difficult to get "face time" or when an informal setting involving personal interaction is required. Given the importance of relationship development in a referral-driven environment, networking is an activity that should be carefully planned rather than implemented on the fly.

Advertising

Advertising refers to any paid form of nonpersonal presentation and promotion of ideas, goods or services by an identifiable sponsor, typically using mass media as the communication vehicle. Common types of mass media vehicles for disseminating advertisements include electronic forms such as radio and television and print forms such as newspapers and magazines. These examples typically represent high-end forms of advertising and are relatively expensive. "Big media" such as radio and television carries a big price tag and tends to "hog" the marketing budget. A third but less significant category includes outdoor and display advertising. The following paragraphs present important considerations with regard to media options. (Box 9.1 lists the categories of advertising approaches.) More detail on print and electronic media is presented later.

Unfortunately, in the past many in healthcare have equated marketing with advertising. Not only has this created a distorted perception of the nature of marketing, but it has placed undue emphasis on the most expensive form of promotions.

Box 9.1 Advertising options

- Print
    Newspapers
    Magazines
    Journals
    Newsletters
    Brochures/flyers
- Electronic
    Television
    Radio
    Internet
- Outdoor
    Billboards
    Transportation venues
- Display
    Store displays
    Posters

Personal Selling

Personal selling involves the oral presentation of information through a conversation with one or more prospective purchasers with the objective of making a sale. The primary purposes of personal selling are to: (1) find prospects; (2) convince prospects to buy the product; and (3) keep existing customers satisfied. Personal sales not only includes formal sales calls but also takes place at health fairs, trade shows and other public venues.

With personal sales the message can be refined or explained in greater detail to correct any misunderstandings or difficulties that the receiver had. Personal selling also has an advantage over advertising in that it provides more direct control over who receives the message. With personal selling, a company can directly target the audience for its communications. Personal sales also provides the opportunity for direct feedback from customers, allowing the salesperson to serve as the eyes and ears of the organization.

Well-established personal selling activities in healthcare include calls on physicians by pharmaceutical and medical supplier representatives, calls on consumers by insurance salesmen, and calls on hospitals by biomedical equipment representatives. More recently, healthcare providers have become active in personal sales, with hospital representatives calling on referring physicians, employers, and other organizations to promote the hospital's emergency room, sports medicine program, or a particular service line.

Personal selling carries a high price tag, with expenses for a sales staff, travel, and technical and equipment support. The number of sales calls a person can make in one day is limited, and sales calls to referral physician offices or companies are time-consuming.

Sales Promotion

Sales promotion refers to any activity or material that acts as a direct inducement by offering added value to or incentive for resellers, salespersons or consumers to achieve a specific sales and marketing objective. Some "pull" incentives used with consumer health products include: money off next purchase, cash refunds, discount coupons, buy-one-get-more-free promotions, consumer contests, loyalty cards, free trials (i.e., samples), free products, price reductions, merchandising and point-of-sale displays, and advertising in stores. A "push" strategy is implemented by pharmaceutical representatives when they leave samples at physicians' offices. The idea is that the physician will "push" the product through the channel to the end consumer.

Exhibiting at trade shows, professional meetings and conferences is also a means of sales promotion. This provides an opportunity to expose the organization or product to hard-to-reach prospects such as physicians or hospital administrators. While it may be almost impossible to get past the gatekeepers at the doctor's office to make a pitch, the exhibition hall brings the doctor right to your booth. The decision to exhibit and the type of exhibit that is developed depends on the nature of the organization and the product as well as the characteristics of the target audience.

Direct Marketing

Direct marketing involves an interactive system of marketing that uses one or more advertising media to effect a measurable response and/or transaction. The main difference between direct marketing and other forms of promotion is that the marketer can directly target an audience to deliver a message that appeals to its specific needs.

Direct mail is a form of direct marketing whereby selected customers are sent advertising material addressed specifically to them and often customized to reflect their interests. This has been traditionally done through the postal service, but more contemporary approaches use fax or e-mail transmission. Everyone is familiar with the "junk mail" that regularly turns up in the mailbox. This is now being joined by unsolicited faxes and "spam" e-mail messages.

Despite the annoyance that these types of solicitations cause for many people, they are nevertheless considered effective marketing tools. Marketers like direct mail because it can be highly targeted and personalized and can make use creative designs and formats. Even with a two percent response rate, marketers find direct mail to be reasonably cost effective. Research has shown that certain segments of the population are actually relatively responsive to mailed solicitations, and materials related to healthcare are less likely to be summarily discarded than others. *Direct response advertising* involves promotions via print or electronic media that provide a call-in number for potential customers. Typically a toll-free number is provided and individuals who want to order a product or service or to obtain more information are instructed to call this number.

Telemarketing is a form of direct marketing that most people are familiar with and an approach that has generated considerable backlash among consumers. Most people are familiar with outbound telemarketing in which individuals operating from a telephone bank call individuals from a prospect list in order to offer a good or service. This may involve "cold calls" to individuals or households for which the demand for goods and services is unknown. More likely, the telephone numbers that are used as a sampling frame are randomly generated for areas that have the approximate characteristics of the target audience.

A more benign form of telemarketing in healthcare involves periodic contacts with individuals who have expressed an interest to the healthcare organization with regard to a particular program or topic. It is assumed that the individual is willing to receive calls describing such programs and will not consider them an imposition due to their implied previous interest. Hospital call centers frequently use this approach to contact prospects for various services and programs. (Table 9.1 presents a matrix for use in promotion decision making.)

Table 9.1 Matrix for promotional decision making

Promotional Technique	Uses	Audience	Timeframe	Relative Cost	Advantages	Disadvantages
Public relations	Awareness Visibility Service rollout	General public Stakeholders Decision makers Influentials	Short-term within a longer-term strategic context	Primarily staff time with little out-of-pocket costs	Broad reach Low cost Short lead time	Not targeted Short shelf-life
Communication	Awareness Visibility Education Relationship development/ maintenance	General public Stakeholders Existing customers Employees	On-going with periodic flurry of activity	Primarily staff time with moderate out-of-pocket costs	Direct to target Low cost	Narrow focus Staffing costs
Community outreach	Awareness Visibility Education Relationship development/ maintenance	General public Targeted consumer groups	On-going with periodic flurry of activity	Primarily staff time with moderate out-of-pocket costs	On-going presence Personalized Localized	High effort Long lead time
Networking	Awareness Business development Relationship development/ maintenance Intelligence gathering	Key stakeholders Potential partners Potential referrers	On-going	Little additional cost	On-going Targeted	Time commitment

Technique	Exposure	Target	Timeframe	Cost	Advantages	Disadvantages
Direct Marketing	Product introduction Call to action	Targeted consumer groups	Short-term but with some lead time	Moderate cost	Focused Customized Multiple exposures	Low response rate High unit cost Short shelf-life
Personal Sales	Visibility Close contracts Relationship development/maintenance	Influentials Potential customers	Regular, periodic contact	Moderate-to-high cost	Face-to-face On-going Feedback on market	Sales force maintenance Cost
Advertising	Awareness Visibility Image enhancement consumer groups	General public Targeted lead time	Typically long-term with long	High cost Easily targeted	Many options Design options Short shelf-life	Cost Negative connotation

Source: Used with permission from Thomas, Richard K., and Michael Calhoun (2007). *Marketing Matters: A Guide for Healthcare Executives.* Chicago: Health Administration Press, pp. 105–106.

Box 9.2 The promotional mix: a case study

A hospital introducing a new "open" MRI (magnetic resonance imaging) option might use the following mix of promotional efforts (with the category in parentheses):

- Press releases (public relations)
- Open house (public relations)
- Brochure distribution (public relations)
- Sales calls on referring physicians (personal selling)
- Radio commercials (advertising)
- Contacting existing patients (customer relationship management)

Telemarketing is more expensive than direct mail initiatives, but the costs are not unreasonable. Wages for telemarketers are relatively low, and the benefits to a healthcare organization that attracts a new patient are likely to be significant. Obviously, not all healthcare products lend themselves to this approach but a surprising number do.

The Internet has become a virtual marketplace attracting a wide range of buyers and sellers of healthcare products. A variety of healthcare products are now available via the Internet and aggressive e-mail marketing techniques have carried these messages to the desktop of healthcare consumers who frequently turn to the Internet as a first resort when in comes to locating and pricing consumer health products. (Box 9.2 provides an example of the promotional mix for a particular marketing initiative.)

Selecting Among Media Options

Advertising and certain other promotional opportunities typically use some form of media for communication, and a critical part of any marketing plan will be the media plan. The media plan specifies the objectives of the advertising campaign, the target audience, and the media vehicles that will be used to reach that audience. For our discussion, the media are divided into the categories of print media, electronic media, outdoor and display advertising and a residual category of other methods.

Print Media

Print media are the most traditional of the media and can take a variety of forms. *Magazines* are periodical publications that typically carry advertising. These include magazines aimed at the general public as well as "trade" publications geared to the interests of health professionals. There are also a number of consumer-oriented health-related publications produced today.

The advantages of magazine advertising include: (1) opportunity for color reproduction; (2) suitable editorial environment; (3) ability to target best prospects; (4) advertisements are expected by readers; (5) long life spans; (6) read at leisure; and (7) potentially high readership. The disadvantages of magazine advertising include: (1) ads positioned in "desert" areas seldom noticed by readers; (2) ads lost in the "clutter" of the magazine; and (3) their infrequent publication. Magazine advertising has the potential to be cost effective, depending on the audience served.

Newspapers include weekly and daily news publications. These can be national, regional or local in their distribution. Newspaper advertising has the advantages of: (1) extensive coverage volume; (2) flexibility in terms of timing; and (3) the use of illustrations. The disadvantages include: (1) an untargeted method of reaching the intended audience; and (2) difficulty in getting people to notice the advertising content. Depending on the market, newspaper advertising can be relatively expensive, making it important to match the marketing objectives with the benefits of this medium.

Most cities now have *"alternative" newspapers*, usually weeklies that have emerged to cover aspects of the news thought to be neglected by the mainstream press. In some communities, readership of alternative newspapers approximates that of the conventional press, making them appropriate vehicles for the advertising of many healthcare products. They are particularly suited for the promotion of "progressive" or innovative healthcare services that are likely to appeal to a population interested in holistic medicine or alternative therapies.

Many communities have spawned *special interest newspapers* devoted to some aspect of health. Some areas produce regular healthcare newspapers that chronicle developments in the local healthcare arena. Other types of newspapers have become available devoted to health, such as those dealing with fitness and wellness, sports, and alternative therapies. These could represent advertising venues for a range of goods and services.

Professional *journals* are possibly more ubiquitous in healthcare than in any other industry, with physicians and other health professionals exposed to a wide range of professional publications. Some of these are academically oriented and typically do not carry advertisements. However, even mainstream medical journals like the *Journal of the American Medical Association* and the *New England Journal of Medicine* carry advertisements. Pharmaceutical companies are heavy advertisers in these publications as are medical supply, equipment and information technology vendors.

Newsletters have also become a common source of information in healthcare. Due to the rapid changes that occur in the industry, the lead time required for more traditional publications means they cannot accommodate the needs of an industry in transition. Newsletters, thus, have become a valuable source of current information. While advertising opportunities are rare in newsletters, the vehicles do provide a venue for publicizing new programs, services or organizational changes. The emergence of electronic newsletters has revolutionized the newsletter publishing enterprise.

Directories have become an increasingly important means of gaining visibility for healthcare organizations. The telephone Yellow Pages is a well known directory, and healthcare organizations spend significant amounts for listings in this directory. Some directories are compiled for bureaucratic record-keeping purposes, such as state physician directories or the hospital association's hospital directory. These are not generally intended for commercial use, and an organization's inclusion may or may not be mandatory. Some directories are compiled for administrative purposes but shared with a larger audience.

Another category of directories is those that are commercially produced for distribution. One function of these is to provide visibility to the organizations that are listed. There may be fees for listing the organization and the directories are typically sold to customers who need the information. Thus, there may be directories of physicians, hospitals, information technology vendors, and so forth. A number of publishers compile and distribute directories as their primary business activity. An increasing number of directories are being posted on the Internet.

Electronic Media

Electronic media have become the promotional venue *du jour* as new opportunities have arisen to supplement traditional advertising channels. Obviously a more contemporary format than traditional print media, electronic media include television (and its derivatives), radio, cinema and now the Internet. *Television* is often the first advertising medium that comes to mind and it does have several advantages. These include: (1) the ability to build a high level of awareness; (2) access to large audiences; (3) the ability to demonstrate a product (using sound and vision); (4) compulsiveness; and (5) a comfortable, at-home viewing environment. The disadvantages include the fact that commercial breaks may be seen as irritating, the medium is considered to be transient, and the audience cannot be very targeted. In addition, television advertising time is very expensive.

Historically, television advertising concentrated on the national networks. However, with the advent of cable television and satellite broadcasting, that situation has changed. The fragmentation of viewers has resulted in the development of homogenous groups that support particular cable channels. This makes it possible to target the television audience much more precisely. Further, satellite television subscribers are likely to be upscale innovators if that is the type of population that is being sought. Advertising time is much less expensive in these venues than on network television.

Radio is a longstanding advertising medium that has a lot of advantages. Radios are often considered as "companions" more so than television and other electronic forms. The most important attribute is the ability to precisely target the audience, not only with regard to the station but even with time of day. On the other hand, radio has the disadvantages of lacking visual attributes, being a transient medium, and having a small audience. Radio advertising time is relatively inexpensive, especially compared to television advertising, and production costs are certainly lower. (Box 9.3 describes the "informercial" form of promotions.)

Box 9.3 The healthcare "infomercial"

The growth of electronic media has spawned a new form of advertisement that is often favored by healthcare organizations, the "infomercial". Infomercials may take the form of 15–60 minute television or radio commercials typically presented in a casual talk show format that is designed to look like an ordinary television program. These may also be presented in a standard 30–60 second commercial format. The infomercial is framed as an educational piece and the sponsor is unobtrusively referenced. The intent is to soft sell the organization or service by giving the impression that they sponsor is the authority on that topic, thus attracting customers without having to overtly solicit them. Physicians or other health experts may be drafted to present the material.

Over the past several years, an explosion has occurred in *Internet* advertising. This does not refer to marketing websites (to be discussed later) but to the placement of banners and pop-up advertisements on existing websites. Since the advent of the Internet age, growing numbers of healthcare organizations have begun advertising on web sites. The majority of these have been consumer health products companies, but some providers are also advertising on the World Wide Web. This is particularly true for providers offering elective services (e.g., laser eye surgery) who need to drive potential business to their doors.

In addition to banners and pop-up ads, many healthcare organizations are paying a fee to be listed on various Internet-based directories of physicians, hospitals or other providers. Although the effectiveness of this form of marketing has not been thoroughly documented, there appears to be continued interest among healthcare organizations in maintaining some advertising on Internet sites.

Another form of media involves display advertising in the form of outdoor advertising, transportation advertising, and posters. Outdoor advertising involves primarily billboards although other types of signage (e.g., banners, portable signs) might be utilized. While billboard advertising has its critics, it appears to be surprisingly popular with healthcare organizations such as hospitals, health plans, and voluntary associations. Transportation or transit advertising would involve ads placed on buses, taxis, and other commercial vehicles (e.g., trucks, business cars). Posters are signs that are displayed in public places in order to attract attention to the organization, service or event.

The advantages of this type of display advertising are its (1) ability to build high awareness levels; (2) exposure to large numbers of people; (3) relatively low costs, (4) short- and long-term possibilities; (5) opportunity for national campaigns; and (6) segmentation possibilities. The disadvantages of this type of advertising include: (1) it may be subject to the effect of weather; (2) some sites are subject to environmental criticism; and (3) the general low regard that outdoor advertising is held in by much of the public (Table 9.2 offers guidelines for media decision making).

Table 9.2 Matrix for media decision making

Medium	Uses	Audience	Resource requirements	Relative cost	Advantages	Disadvantages
Television	Exposure Service introduction Call to action		Production skills Creative skills	High	Consumer appeal Multiple exposures	Cost Negative connotation Short shelf-life Competing ads
Network		General public			Broad reach	Diffuse impact
Cable		Targeted consumers			Targeted	Narrow impact
Radio	Exposure Service introduction Call to action	General public/targeted	Production skills Creative skills	Moderate	Broad or narrow	Cost Short shelf-life
Newspapers	Exposure Service introduction Call to action	General public		Moderate	Broad reach Low unit cost Frequent exposure	Cost Competing ads Short shelf-life
Magazines	Exposure Service introduction Call to action	General public (but higher end)		Moderate	Moderate shelf-life Design options	Cost Competing ads
Internet	Education Channel business Relationship development/maintenance	General public Targeted consumer groups		Low	Appealing medium Interactive	Incomplete coverage Spam annoyance On-going

Source: Used with permission from Thomas, Richard K., and Michael Calhoun (2007). *Marketing Matters: A Guide for Healthcare Executives*. Chicago: Health Administration Press, p. 107.

Criteria for Selecting Promotional Techniques

There are a number of factors to be considered when selecting among promotional options. Factors such as context, message, channel and timing should all be considered.

Context

The context (or environment) is the situation in which the communication occurs. It includes the physical context and social context, as well as the number of people involved, the relationships of participants, surrounding events, and potential distractions. The physical location could be the receiver's home, the workplace, the physician's office, or any number of other physical settings. Factors such as temperature, the time of day, nearby people, and any concurrent activities all contribute to the establishment of the physical context.

The social context may take the form of a group of friends, work associates, or even strangers. The social context may be familiar or strange and will influence the level of formality, use of language, familiarity with the audience members, use of humor, content of the message, appropriate dress, and many other factors.

The context for the promotion of a healthcare product is an important consideration. The same information conveyed by the physician in his/her office, around the water fountain at work, by a close family member, or via the Internet will have different degrees of impact. Some contexts are clearly more conducive to the promotion of healthcare ideas, organizations and products than others.

Message

The message represents the information that is transmitted from the marketer to the target audience. This constitutes the content of the promotional piece and addresses the issues of what to say and how to say it. The message will include the explanation, response options, set of instructions, and/or recommendations to be conveyed to the audience. The marketer must determine what information is to be provided, the style and tone in which it is to be presented, and the information that the message must ultimately convey. If the message does not resonate with the target audience, the promotional effort is likely to fail.

Issues discussed above – such as the nature of the product, community standards, and the characteristics of the target audience – all should be taken into consideration when crafting the message. A separate "industry" has developed focusing on the type of content that resonates with different population segments.

Channels

Marketing messages are conveyed through a specific channel or channels. Channels are also referred to as the medium, hence references to "mass media" or to "the media." The channel determines the means by which the message is delivered and received. Channels differ from each other in terms of attributes, attention getting, and volume of information conveyed, among other factors. A book, for example, has more credibility than television but is less attention getting. More information can be communicated in a newspaper article than a television newscast. On the other hand, television has live pictures that make the communication more engaging.

The variety of channel options has increased dramatically in recent years, creating both an opportunity and a challenge for marketers. Population segments vary widely in their preferences for communication channels, and detailed information is available on which segments of the population prefer to receive their health-related information form radio, newspapers, the Internet or their health plan, for example. (Box 9.4 provides questions to ask when selecting a channel for communication.)

Box 9.4 Selecting the appropriate channel

Each type of channel has benefits and drawbacks. Factors to be considered (and questions to be asked) include:

- The intended audience(s)
  - Will the channel reach and influence the intended audiences?
  - Is the channel acceptable to and trusted by the intended audiences?
- Compatibility with the message
  - Is the channel appropriate for conveying information at the desired level of simplicity or complexity?
  - Is the tone of the channel compatible with the nature of the message being conveyed?
  - If skills need to be modeled, can the channel model and demonstrate specific behaviors?
- Channel reach
  - How many people will be exposed to the message through this channel?
  - Can the channel meet intended audience interaction needs?
  - Can the channel allow the intended audience to control the pace of information delivery?
- Cost and accessibility
  - Is this a cost-effective channel given the objectives?
  - Are the resources available to use the channel in the manner intended?
- Activities and materials:
  - Is the channel appropriate for the activity or material you plan to produce?
  - Will the channel reinforce the message being delivered through other routes?

Timing

People use the expression: "Timing is everything," and that certainly applies to marketing. Timing can be thought of in a variety of ways. In a mechanical sense, timing could refer to the day of the week or time of the day at which the promotional message is delivered. It could also refer to the frequency of exposures established. Radio and television advertising is carefully planned to take advantage of the habits of listeners or viewers, and information is available on the timing that is appropriate for various target audiences.

Timing may also refer to the state of readiness on the part of the target audience vis-à-vis the message that is being conveyed. Different audiences are amenable to the receipt of information at different times, not in terms of clock time but in terms of their current situation. It is very difficult, for example, to interest teenagers or young adults in the risk of chronic disease since their age and health status make this an irrelevant topic. Or a woman may only be interested in information on pediatricians around the time that her baby is due to be delivered. It is very difficult to talk about HIV and AIDS within some church settings, and this type of situation is a particular issue in social marketing, since many topics are unpleasant or make the recipient uncomfortable due to their state of readiness. (Box 9.5 illustrates different stages of communication readiness.)

Box 9.5 Stages of readiness

Members of the target audience (or whole population segments for that matter) are likely to display various states of readiness when it comes to marketing. Consumers might be considered to be at one of the following stages of readiness:

- Unaware of the situation (that the service might address)
- Aware of the existence of the situation but does not personality identify with it.
- Concedes acceptance of the situation but does not define it as a threat
- Perceives as a threat but is not motivated to take action
- Motivated to take action and ready to receive the message

Chapter 10
Social Marketing

Social marketing has become increasingly important in healthcare as public health entities and not-for-profit organizations have attempted to promote services to their target audiences. Even for-profit healthcare organizations may have occasion to utilize social marketing techniques. While social marketing utilizes many of the methods employed by traditional marketers, significant differences exist. This chapter provides an introduction to social marketing, describes some of the techniques that have been adopted by social marketers, and explains the importance of health communication for this endeavor.

What is Social Marketing?

"Social marketing" in healthcare can be defined as the application of commercial marketing techniques to the development and implementation of programs that influence the attitudes, knowledge, and behavior of target audiences in the direction of improving individual and community health status.

Social marketing was "born" as a discipline in the 1970s, when marketing professionals realized that the same marketing principles that were being used to sell products to consumers could be used to "sell" ideas, attitudes and behaviors. Social marketing, it was argued, differs from other types of marketing only with respect to the objectives of the marketer and his or her organization. Thus, social marketing seeks to influence social behaviors not to benefit the "seller" but to benefit the target audience and the general society.

In contrast to the top-down approach of traditional marketing, social marketers listen to the needs and desires of the target audience and build the marketing campaign from the bottom up. This focus on the consumer, of course, requires in-depth research and constant re-evaluation. To "sell" healthy behavior, social marketing starts with audience research that leads to the segmentation of the target audience into groups with common risk behaviors, motivations, and information channel preferences. The "marketing mix" is continually refined on the basis of consumer feedback.

Since the intent of social marketing is typically not to sell something but to influence knowledge, attitudes and behavior, the approach is different from that of traditional marketing. Instead of a sales pitch, the target audience might be exposed to an "intervention" in, for example, the form of an educational program.

Virtually all Americans have been exposed to health messages through public education campaigns that seek to change the social climate in order to encourage healthy behaviors, create awareness, change attitudes, and motivate individuals to adopt recommended actions. Social marketing campaigns have traditionally relied on mass communication (such as public service announcements on billboards, radio, and television) and educational messages in printed materials (such as pamphlets) to deliver health messages. Other campaigns have integrated mass media with community-based programs such as health fairs.

Social marketing increasingly takes advantage of contemporary technology, such as the Internet, that can target audiences, tailor messages, and engage people in interactive, ongoing exchanges about their health. As population-based approaches to healthcare have become more common, the role of health communication has expanded. Community-centered prevention shifts attention from the individual to group-level change and emphasizes the empowerment of individuals and communities to effect change on multiple levels.

Social marketing can be used for a variety of purposes in healthcare. The functions of social marketing include:

- Increase knowledge and awareness of a health issue, problem, or solution
- Influence perceptions, beliefs, attitudes, and social norms
- Prompt action
- Demonstrate or illustrate skills
- Show the benefits of behavior change
- Increase demand for health services
- Reinforce knowledge, attitudes, or behavior
- Refute myths and misconceptions
- Help coalesce organizational relationships
- Advocate for a health issue or a population group.

The Four P's and Social Marketing

The four P's highlighted in traditional marketing can also be applied, within limits, in social marketing. Here, the "product" may not be a tangible good or even a specific service. A continuum of products exists, ranging from physical products (e.g., condoms) to services (e.g., medical exams), and practices (e.g., breastfeeding), along with more conceptual initiatives (e.g., healthy communities).

"Price" refers to what the consumer must expend in order to obtain the social marketing product, including money, time, effort, or even the risk of embarrassment or disapproval. If the costs, however measured, outweigh the benefits for an individual, the perceived value of the offering will be low, and it will be unlikely to be adopted. However, if the benefits are perceived as greater than their costs, chances of trial and adoption of the product is much greater. Social marketers must balance these considerations, and often end up charging at least a nominal fee to increase perceptions of quality and to confer a sense of "dignity" to the transaction.

In social marketing, "place" may refer to the distribution system or the channels through which consumers are reached with information. This may include doctors' offices, shopping malls, mass media vehicles or in-home demonstrations. With social marketing the physical, social and economic accessibility of the offering and the quality of the service delivery are critical factors. By determining the activities and habits of the target audience, as well as their experience and satisfaction with the existing delivery system, researchers can pinpoint the most effective means of disseminating a chosen message.

Social marketers take full advantage of the variety of options for "promotions" that are available. They may utilize public relations, advertising (including public service announcements), and community outreach as well as other means of promotion. Direct sales may be employed in the form of counselors. Social marketers may also embark on advocacy campaigns that attempt to influence public policy. (Box 10.1 describes a marketing mix strategy for social marketing.)

Social marketing is different, however, and it is felt that additional P's might be added because of the unique nature of social marketing. According to Weinreich (1999), these additional P's should be taken into consideration when it comes to social marketing:

Publics: Social marketers often have many different audiences that their program has to address in order to be successful. "Publics" refers to both the external and internal groups involved in the program. External publics include the target audience, secondary audiences, policymakers, and gatekeepers, while the internal publics are those who are involved in some way with either approval or implementation of the program.

Partnership: Social and health issues are often so complex that one agency cannot effect change by itself. Collaboration among organizations within the community may be required. You need to figure out which organizations have similar goals to yours – not necessarily the same goals – and identify ways you can work together.

Policy: Social marketing programs can do well in motivating individual behavior change, but that is difficult to sustain unless the environment they're in supports that change for the long run. Often, policy change is needed, and media advocacy programs can be an effective complement to a social marketing program.

Steps in the Social Marketing Process

Social marketing shares much with traditional marketing although some allowance must be made for the uniqueness of healthcare. The following paragraphs outline the steps involved in a social marketing initiative.

Box 10.1 A marketing mix strategy for a social marketing campaign

The marketing mix strategy for a breast cancer screening campaign for older women might involve the following elements:

- The *product* could be any of these three behaviors: getting an annual mammogram, seeing a physician each year for a breast exam, and performing monthly breast self-exams.
- The *price* of engaging in these behaviors includes the monetary costs of the mammogram or office visit, potential discomfort and/or embarrassment, time and even the possibility of a "positive" finding.
- The *place* that these medical and educational services are offered might be a mobile van, local hospital clinic worksite depending upon the needs of the target audience.
- *Promotion* could be done through public service announcements, billboards, mass mailings, media events, and community outreach.
- The *"publics"* you might need to address include your target audience (e.g., low-income women aged 40–65), the people who influence their decisions like their husbands or physicians, policymakers, public service directors at local radio stations, as well as your board of directors and office staff.
- *Partnerships* could be cultivated with local or national women's groups, corporate sponsors, medical organizations, service clubs, or media outlets.
- The *policy* aspects of the campaign might focus on increasing access to mammograms through lower costs, requiring insurance and Medicaid coverage of mammograms, or increasing federal funding for breast cancer research.

Each element of the marketing mix should be taken into consideration as the program is developed. Marketing research should be employed to finalize the attributes of product, price, place, promotion, and related attributes.

Source: http://www.social-marketing.com/Whatis.html

Identifying Who Must Act to Solve the Problem

- Collect and analyze demographic, socioeconomic, cultural and other data on the target audience
- Select target segments for the program
- Profile the targeted segments in terms of relevant attributes
- Identify those in a position to change conditions under which the targeted behaviors occur
- Identify the specific partners that need to be involved

Conducting Formative Research

- Understand selected target segment: needs, wants, hopes, fears, knowledge, attitude, behavior, perceived risk
- For the targeted group determine their readiness for changing in the targeted behaviors
- Determine the environments, situations, or settings in which the targeted behavior occurs
- Research behavioral determinants of the desired behavior for the selected target segment
- Plan initial concepts and program elements

Designing the Project

- Set behavioral objectives for the target audience
- Design interventions for the target audience
- Apply marketing principles (the "marketing mix")
- Pretest all products, services and messages including interventions

Delivering and Monitoring the Program

- Train and motivate front-line staff
- Build products/programs and distribute/execute them
- Distribute materials
- Refine product/program and materials as midcourse monitoring data suggest
- Sustain the effort long enough to make a difference

Conducting Evaluation

- Conduct process and outcome evaluation
- Revise implementation plans and models in accordance with program changes

    (Box 10.2 descusses the role of change agents in social marketing.)

Health Communication

Any discussion of social marketing needs to consider the issue of health communication. Communication refers to the transmission or exchange of information and implies the sharing of meaning among those who are communicating. Health communication encompasses the study and use of communication strategies to inform

Box 10.2 Change agents

Social marketers should identify any potential agents for change that may be particularly helpful in reaching different target groups. These could include:

1. Connectors (those who link): how will we identify and involve those who can spread the message of the campaign through their networks? Who knows lots of people in the targeted groups and can get messages to them?
2. Mavens (those who know/teach): how will we identify and involve those who can and will provide needed knowledge to those implementing the campaign's components? Who is in a position to share knowledge relevant to the issue? Who are the trendsetters and early adopters of related practices?
3. Persuaders (those who motivate): how will we identify and involve those who can motivate others to adopt the behaviors sought by the campaign? Who has a passion for the issue/goal and who can reach the target audience? Who has the energy, enthusiasm, likeability, optimism, and trustworthiness to reach the targeted audiences?

and influence individual and community knowledge, attitudes and practices (KAP) with regard to health and healthcare. (Box 10.3 discusses the implications of low health literacy for social marketing)

Health communication can take place on a number of different levels, and the Centers for Disease Control and Prevention (U.S. office of Disease Prevention and Health Promotion, 2004) have identified the following levels of impact:

The individual: The individual is the most fundamental target for health-related change, since it is individual behaviors that affect health status. Communication can affect the individual's awareness, knowledge, attitudes, self-efficacy, and skills for behavior change. Activity at all other levels ultimately aims to affect and support individual change.

The social network: An individual's relationships and the groups to which an individual belongs can have a significant impact on his or her health. Health communication programs can work to shape the information a group receives and may attempt to change communication patterns or content. Opinion leaders within a network are often a point of entry for health programs.

Organizations: Organizations include formal groups with a defined structure, such as associations, clubs, and civic groups; worksites; schools; primary healthcare settings; and retailers. Organizations can carry health messages to their membership, provide support for individual efforts, and make policy changes that enable individual change.

Communities: The collective well-being of communities can be fostered by creating structures and policies that support healthy lifestyles and by reducing or eliminating hazards in social and physical environments. Community-level initiatives are planned

Box 10.3 Health literacy and social marketing

The literacy level of any target audience must be taken into consideration. *Health literacy* is defined as the ability to read, understand, and act on health information. People of any age, income, race, or background can find it challenging to understand health information. Low health literacy has been identified as a serious barrier to health communication. The health literacy problem represents a crisis of understanding medical information rather than one of access to information. In fact, the health of 90 million people in the United States may be at risk because of the difficulty some patients experience in understanding and acting on health information.

Medical information is becoming increasingly complex and, all too frequently, physicians do not explain this information in layperson's terms or in a way that patients can understand. Physicians are under increasing time pressure in today's clinical setting, and they may not even be aware when patients do not understand medical information or instructions. When this occurs, a crucial part of their medical care is missing, sometimes resulting in adverse clinical outcomes.

The inability to read, understand, and act on health information is an emerging public health communication issue that affects people of all ages, races, and income levels. Research shows that most consumers need help understanding healthcare information. Regardless of reading level, patients prefer medical information that is easy to read and understand. For people who don't have strong reading skills, however, easy-to-read healthcare materials are essential.

Limited health literacy increases the disparity in healthcare access among exceptionally vulnerable populations (such as racial/ethnic minorities and the elderly). Low health literacy is an enormous cost burden for the American healthcare system. Annual healthcare costs for individuals with low literacy skills are four times higher than those with higher literacy skills. Problems with patient compliance and medical errors may be based on poor understanding of health information. The fact that only about 50% of all patients take medications as directed illustrates the downside of low health literacy.

Patients with low health literacy and chronic diseases, such as diabetes, asthma, or hypertension, have less knowledge of their disease and its treatment and fewer correct self-management skills than literate patients. Patients with low literacy skills face a 50% increased risk of hospitalization, compared with patients who had adequate literacy skills. These statistics reflect the pivotal role played by health communication in addressing individual and community health issues.

and led by organizations and institutions that can influence health, such as schools, worksites, healthcare settings, community groups, and government agencies.

Society: Society as a whole has many influences on individual behavior, including norms and values, attitudes and opinions, laws and policies, and the physical, economic, cultural, and information environments. Some policies implemented though agencies of the federal government have had an impact on health indicators.

Clearly, the more levels a communication program can influence, the greater the likelihood of creating and sustaining the desired change. Social marketing alone, however, cannot change systemic problems related to health, such as poverty, environmental degradation, or lack of access to healthcare. Well-designed health communication activities, however, can help individuals better understand their own and their communities' needs so that they can take appropriate actions to maximize health.

References

U.S. Office of Disease Prevention and Health Promotion (2004). "Health Communication," *Healthy People 2010* (vol. 1). Washington, DC: U.S. Government Printing Office.
Weinreich, Nedra Kline (1999). *Hands-On Social Marketing: A Step-by-Step Guide.* Thousand Oaks, CA: Sage.

Chapter 11
The New Healthcare Marketing

Recent developments in healthcare have created a need for innovative marketing techniques. Indeed, the nature of marketing has changed greatly during the past two decades. The 1990s witnessed the adoption of techniques from other industries and the development of new healthcare-specific approaches. This chapter describes the implications of these changes for healthcare marketing and indicates how new approaches such as customer relationship management, direct-to-consumer marketing and business-to-business marketing fit into the healthcare marketing picture.

Trends Driving the New Marketing

Over the past decade healthcare has experienced a number of trends related to marketing that have dramatically altered the marketing landscape. These include the following:

From a mass marketing approach to a more targeted approach. Although most industries were moving away from a mass marketing approach by the time healthcare jumped on the marketing bandwagon, healthcare organizations initially adopted approaches that emphasized the transmission of a uniform message to the general public. This involved the use of mass media that broadcast to an undifferentiated audience. Eventually, health professionals learned that this was not an efficient means of reaching their potential customers and subsequently adopted more targeted approaches to getting their message out.

From image marketing to service marketing. As marketing became more accepted, healthcare organizations – most notably hospitals – emphasized the marketing of their image rather than specific services. This was the era of "all things to all people" and "one size fits all," and the focus was on enhancing the overall visibility and reputation of the organization. As it became obvious that neither of these catch-phrases was realistic, the emphasis began to shift to service marketing, with a specific service being promoted to specific target audiences.

From one-size-fits-all to personalization and customization. As indicated by the above, early marketing efforts by healthcare organizations emphasized the delivery of a standardized message to an undifferentiated audience. Ultimately, it became clear that not all consumers were candidates for all services and that this approach tended to "water down" the impact. At the same time, the importance of the consumer was being rediscovered and, assisted by modern technology, it became important to not only target high priority audiences but to customize the message to meet their unique needs.

From an emphasis on the healthcare episode to one on the long-term relationship. Emulating marketers in other industries, much early healthcare marketing focused on "making the sale." The goal was to drive business to the organization even if it was for a one-time purchase. Ultimately, it became obvious that healthcare consumers were different from other consumers, and the nature of the service provided demanded a different type of relationship (not to mention the lifetime value of a loyal healthcare customer). Relationship marketing emerged as a means of getting closer to the customer by developing a long-term association through careful attention to customer needs and service delivery. This represents a departure from the traditional approach in healthcare in which the focus was on capturing the discrete episode of care.

From market "ignorance" to market intelligence. Early marketing efforts in healthcare were carried out from a position of ignorance. Until the 1980s there was no need to identify the market for health services much less profile its characteristics. A patient was a patient from the standpoint of the traditional healthcare administrator and knowing more about the patient (and his environment) was not considered a worthwhile effort. As the market became more competitive and consumerism emerged in healthcare, it became not only important but critical that healthcare organizations knew a lot about their consumers.

From low tech to high tech. Although the healthcare industry has lagged behind other industries in terms of the adoption of information technology, the new healthcare marketing is making increasing use of contemporary technology. The need to better target increasingly narrower segments of the population, integrate data from disparate sources and support increasingly complex relationships with customers, coupled with advances in technology, have encouraged the development of direct-to-consumer marketing, customer relationship management, and Web-based marketing.

Emerging Marketing Techniques

The marketing techniques that appear to be gaining momentum in healthcare can be divided into those that involve organizational changes and those that are technology based. The former category implies an innovative approach at a conceptual level and the latter the use of technology to modify an existing technique or the creation of innovative technology-based marketing techniques.

Leveraging the Organization

The techniques described below illustrate how healthcare organizations are taking organizationally based approaches to enhancing their marketing capabilities.

Business-to-Business Marketing

Business-to-business marketing is nothing new in healthcare. Healthcare organizations have long been major purchasers of a wide variety of goods, and an increasing amount of marketing in healthcare involves business-to-business transactions. The increasing corporatization of healthcare means that more and more relationships are between one corporate body and another. The traditional doctor–patient relationship has been supplanted by contractual arrangements between groups of buyers and sellers of health services. Many hospital programs now target corporate customers rather than individual patients.

Business-to-business marketing involves building profitable, value-oriented relationships between two businesses and the individuals within them. Business marketers focus on a few customers, with usually much larger, more complex and technically oriented sales processes. Statistical tools, data mining techniques, and other sorts of research that work so well in the land of consumer marketing must be adapted to the needs of the business-to-business marketer. B2B purchases are often a considered, group decision while decisions made by consumers are more personal and impulsive.

The most common technique for business-to-business marketing in healthcare is personal sales. Whether we are talking about health plans marketing to major employers, medical supply vendors marketing to hospitals, or hospitals marketing to business coalitions, there is an emphasis on face-to-face promotional techniques. Personal sales is supplemented by public relations, sales promotion and advertising.

A number of factors might be thought to contribute to successful B2B marketing efforts. This obviously starts with a good product that is well positioned and exhibits a unique selling proposition. B2B sales should focus on relationship development rather than short-term gains, emphasizing the service component of the relationship. Those organizations successful at B2B marketing often present themselves as "consultants" rather than sales representatives. (Box 11.1 discusses co. marketing opportunities in healthcare.)

Service Line Marketing

Over the past few years service line management has been adopted by hundreds of hospitals nationwide. Hospitals are looking for ways to become more agile, move closer to their customers, strengthen relationships with physicians, become more profitable, and develop more innovative and effective ways to serve their patients.

A service line is a tightly integrated, overlapping network of semiautonomous clinical services and a business enterprise that bundles needed resources to provide specialized, focused care to a patient population. The most common service lines include cardiovascular services, orthopedics, rehabilitation, women's services, children's services, and oncology services. Service lines can be "virtual" in that all components are not under one roof. Some services are horizontal and cross departments and disciplines. Indeed, the focus in not on the facility, but on the services. A service line may be created around a business that is already well established, or the concept can be used to focus on a new service or niche.

The service line platform integrates clinical and support services on a matrix management grid to create the horizontal integration of clinical services along a traditional continuum of care and the vertical integration of support services. Also built into this platform are education and wellness programs, retail models, business development functions, and physician relationship development.

This approach facilitates the marketing of services in many ways, and the close relationship that can develop between operations and marketing represents an advantage. In fact, many such efforts have been criticized for being *primarily* marketing initiatives. The focusing of marketing resources in this manner does have its benefits. While it is encouraging that so much faith is placed in the marketing function, the same caveats apply here as elsewhere. To wit, marketing is wasted effort if the service line is not well developed and well managed, if service can not be efficiently provided, and if mechanisms are not in place for measuring the impact of the marketing effort.

Whether the service line concept is an effective approach to healthcare strategy development is still open to debate, and little hard evidence documents the merits of this approach. There is some question as to the significance of service lines to customers. Ideally, service lines are designed to address consumer needs. However, it could be argued that most consumers do not think about healthcare in terms of vertical silos of care, but as a continuum of services that extend across clinical lines. As service lines become more entrenched in healthcare a better understanding of their meaning for consumers should be established.

Internal Marketing

Internal marketing refers to efforts by a service provider to effectively train and motivate its customer-contact employees and other supporting service people to work as a team to generate customer satisfaction. Internal marketing represents a marketing effort, inside a company's four walls, that targets internal audiences. Its goal is to increase communications among staff members so that a marketing campaign's effectiveness is maximized. It recognizes that people who work together stand in exactly the same relationships to each other as do customers and suppliers.

By redefining employees as valued customers, it is felt that the organization can engender greater commitment to its goals. This in turn will allow the organization to improve the quality of service to its external customers. Internal marketing represents a combination of marketing, human resources, training and behavioral science.

In order for internal marketing to be successful, employees must be made fully aware of the aims and activities of the organization. It is amazing how often employees of large healthcare organizations are unaware of services or programs the organization offers. While this could happen in any organization, it appears to be an inherent characteristic of healthcare organizations. Employees must also be given a basic understanding of the nature of the organization's customers and the manner in which the organization interacts with them.

There is nothing magic about internal marketing; in fact, most of it involves the application of common sense. Among the most common features of internal marketing programs are meetings, special events, company anniversary celebrations, appreciation dinners, brown bag lunches, off-site/satellite offices visits, internal newsletters, bulletin boards, e-mail newsletters, intranets, and broadcast e-mails.

The key to successful internal marketing is effective communication. For whatever reason, healthcare organizations involve numerous barriers to communication. For internal marketing to work, everyone must be kept current on developments and everyone must be able to contribute to the dialogue. Employees who do not feel like they have input into the process are not likely to be become great ambassadors for the organization.

Box 11.1 Co-marketing in healthcare

One of the least expensive and most effective ways to get your brand in front of more people is to join forces with another company. Co-marketing typically involves the execution of supporting advertising, promotion and direct mail events that leverage the equities of both the manufacturer and the retailer to build volume and profits. Co-marketing originated in the packaged goods industry and has since been embraced by marketers in other industries. Many lessons learned from the packaged goods industry can be applied in healthcare, especially given the variety of different healthcare organizations that often has to collaborate on a particular care episode. One advantage of co-marketing for healthcare organizations – especially those that do not have the time to develop marketing expertise on their own – is the ability to benefit from the analytical and marketing resources, the advertising clout, and the promotional resources of "partners" with more marketing expertise.

Co-marketing in healthcare, of course, is not without its obstacles. First of all, organizations involved in co-marketing have to and be willing to share information. Healthcare organizations, however, have historically been unwilling to share data about their customers (assuming of course that they have such data). A more significant issue may be fact that healthcare organizations – even those involved in a joint initiative – may actually have different goals. Unlike the packaged goods industry where all parties are focused on a single outcome, healthcare organizations may actually be pursuing disparate if not incompatible goals.

These obstacles can usually be overcome and a growing number of health professionals see the potential benefit to be derived from the co-marketing their services with like-minded organizations.

Leveraging Technology

Direct-to-Consumer Marketing

During the 1990s direct-to-consumer (DTC) marketing began to emerge as a force in healthcare. DTC marketing involves the promotion of goods and services directly to consumers rather than indirectly through some "middleman." Perhaps the best example of this is the efforts of pharmaceutical companies to market directly to consumers thereby bypassing their traditional target audience, physicians. DTC marketing may make use of direct mail techniques, telemarketing, Internet marketing and direct-response advertising.

The beauty of DTC marketing lies in its ability to target specific segments of the population with customized materials while using the information transfer method that is most suited for that segment. Where appropriate it is even possible to pinpoint prospective customers down to the household level. Although there are limited uses for this level of micromarketing in healthcare, there may be situations (e.g., big donor fundraising) in which being able to pinpoint individuals is advantageous.

Although the Internet has served to give impetus to much of the new attention devoted to individual consumers, the DTC movement has affected other media as well. The most significant changes involve the need to shift away from the traditional channels (and marketing targets) to a much more diverse and dispersed target audience. In addition to the Internet, television and print media have experienced a considerable increase in expenditures. Direct mail appears to be making a comeback as well. While much of this has been driven by the pharmaceutical industry, there is no reason to expect that other parties chasing these same consumers will not follow suit. (Box 11.2 discusses one prerequisite for DTC marketing).

Database Marketing

Database marketing (DBM) is a well-established component of marketing in virtually every industry beside healthcare. Database marketing involves the collection, storage, analysis, and use of information regarding customers and their past purchase behaviors. It involves building a comprehensive database of customer profiles and initiating direct marketing based on these profiles. The resulting direct marketing must be response and outcome oriented to fit the notion of database marketing.

Although patients cannot be treated the same way as customers for hamburgers, potential DBM applications to healthcare are almost unlimited. The complexity of healthcare offers opportunities to those who can develop the structure for capitalizing on them, and the data mining potential from a well-designed customer database is considerable.

Choice-driven programs (e.g., senior affinity programs, new moms programs) are a natural for database marketing. Pharmaceutical companies are already using a version of database marketing for targeting customers in their direct-to-consumer campaigns. Now, health plans are beginning to use this approach for segmenting

Box 11.2 Really getting to know the customer

Developments in healthcare marketing demand that the healthcare marketer be in closer touch with the end-user than at any time in memory. She must ultimately develop an in-depth understanding of the wants, needs and preferences of the various categories of potential customers. She must be able to determine who wants particular products and services and the extent to which a population category wants standardization versus customization. This will require the development of an understanding of consumer characteristics and behaviors down to the household level, as is already being done in other industries.

The need to target large numbers of consumers is likely to encourage a resurgence of interest in psychographics and other consumer profiling methodologies. In the past, if you knew a couple of things about a patient or potential patient (e.g., referring doctor, health plan), not much more was needed. In the future, the ability to contact and subsequently cultivate prospective patients is going to place significant pressure on the marketer (as it already is in the pharmaceutical industry).

This new environment is also likely to put the finishing touches on any one-size-fits-all approach in healthcare. The challenges for the marketer will increase by virtue of having to offer unbundled services to a wide array of potential customers with highly specific needs, rather than offering a bundled program to all customers. Take for example the health plan that has historically offered a "standard" package of benefits to all enrollees. In the past, Employer A with a poorly educated, blue-collar workforce offered the same benefits as Employer B with a highly educated, professional workforce. In the future, the plan being offered to Employer A must reflect the needs of the employees of Employer A and, of necessity, be different from the plan being sold to Employer B. These activities cannot be carried out without an in-depth understanding of existing and potential healthcare customers.

their enrollee populations. Database marketing can be used for cross-selling, upselling, follow-up sales, and so forth.

Overt solicitation may be a turnoff for healthcare consumers but, if these opportunities are approached in the right way, they can be perceived positively by the customer. If a patient registers for an educational program (and gives consent for subsequent contact), this may be perceived as having value by the patient.

Many healthcare organizations promote secondary products (e.g., pediatric services to OB patients), and patient data provide the basis for the bundling of various services to the benefit of the patient. The main concern for many is observance of privacy laws, but this shouldn't be a problem for anyone who really understands the issues.

There are several factors that contribute to successful database marketing efforts. Unquestionably, you have to start with adequate information technology capabilities *and* ample opportunities for the collection of customer data. The organization must be able to profile customers in a meaningful way and have the ability to update the information. At the same time, the customer must be made to feel that the organization is providing a service through its database marketing efforts. The opportunities for cross-selling, upselling, follow-up sales and so forth must be packaged as just that – "opportunities" for your customers.

Customer Relationship Management

Customer relationship management (CRM) represents a natural extension of database marketing. Well thought out and executed CRM programs can generate substantial returns. Healthcare organizations are beginning to recognize the benefits of CRM, and increased spending on CRM activities is predicted. Some of the more common goals of implementing technology-driven customer relationship programs include:

- Improving customer service and satisfaction
- Increasing profitability
- Reducing the number of negative customer experiences
- Allocating resources more efficiently
- Reducing expenses to manage customer interactions
- Attracting and retaining customers and prospects
- Staying in front of customers
- Building stronger relationships over time
- Improving clinical outcomes

Customer relationship management involves the creation of a centralized body of knowledge that interfaces internal customer data with external market data. This integrated data set can be analyzed to determine patterns that are relevant for an understanding of the task at hand. The final step involves converting this knowledge into a communication vehicle that allows the healthcare organization to target relevant prospects and deliver the appropriate message.

CRM supports the same activities as database marketing and then some. At a minimum, the CRM system can support information and referral efforts and the promotion of specific programs. Further, the technique should be useful for promoting cross-selling, upselling, repeat sales and so forth.

Successful CRM efforts require, in addition to the requirements above for database marketing, an understanding of and commitment to the organization's mission and its stated goals. CRM should support "thinking outside the box" and allow the organization to establish a partnership with each customer.

Web-Based Marketing

Recent years have seen a surge of interest in the use of the Internet for a wide range of marketing activities in healthcare. Most hospitals have websites up and running, and some healthcare organizations have actually led the way with regard to certain aspects of on-line marketing. At the same time, significant growth has occurred in the number of consumers who search for healthcare information online. Whether it is a patient or a caregiver, the Internet is used as a resource both before and after visiting the doctor.

Healthcare organizations have progressed through the various stages of Internet marketing, moving from the "brochure" stage to information and referral to interactive sites to transactional sites. A smaller number of health systems are pushing customized health information and medical records out to consumers, allowing e-mail communication with physicians and doing some level of actual disease management online.

Healthcare marketers are successfully using off-line techniques to draw consumers into their sites to search for information or respond to specific offers – such as finding a physician, viewing an infant photo, or signing up for a health screening. Once consumers are on line, healthcare organizations are converting these "browsers" into prospects by capturing personal information in a customer database and having them sign up for interactive health news and medical reminders. This allows the hospital to continue to market to them in a more personal way than just advertising on television or through the mail. (The various mistakes that can be made by healthcare organizations in developing websites are described in Box 11.3.)

While Internet marketing might be thought of as a technique in its own right, it really embodies a number of different marketing techniques. The website can serve as a public relations tool by providing information to the general public or key constituencies. It can support community outreach and be a tool for information-and-referral activities. It provides a platform for direct marketing activities as well as serving as the foundation for customer relationship development. Increasingly, healthcare-related sites serve as a platform for direct sales.

Limitations to Contemporary Marketing Techniques

The various contemporary approaches to marketing clearly have useful applications to healthcare. However, there are some barriers to the incorporation of some of the more innovative and technology-based techniques. Quite often, healthcare organizations do not have the personnel or technical resources to implement such techniques. They may lack the information technology infrastructure and often cannot access data in the manner necessary to support some of these techniques. They are not likely to have the know-how to implement database marketing or customer relationship management without bringing in outside consultants.

When it comes to data, not only is the necessary data often lacking, but there are always concerns about the confidentiality of the patient data utilized for some of these techniques. The enactment of HIPAA legislation has made many healthcare organizations gun-shy even when it comes to legitimate uses of personal health data. These concerns are reinforced by questions raised about the appropriateness of using patient data in this manner. The conservative nature of health professionals

Box 11.3 Common web-marketing mistakes

Most healthcare organizations have limited experience with marketing, and this lack of experience is often reflected in their attempts to implement innovative marketing initiatives such as websites. Common web marketing mistakes can be grouped into several different categories. These include:

Failure to adequately plan for the project. The most common mistakes made by healthcare organizations are not having specific objectives or goals from the start and not having a formal plan or strategy.

Making faulty assumptions about customer wants/needs. Healthcare organizations often make assumptions about what site visitors want without really understanding their needs and motivations. This often involves a failure to research on the front end the types of functionality that the site will need. This approach often leads to an "if we build it they'll come" attitude that almost assures failure.

Entrusting the process to inappropriate parties. Another major mistake involves assigning Web site development to inappropriate parties. The inappropriate party could be marketing, information systems, or an enthusiastic employee who is really into the Internet. This might also include choosing a Web developer because he is cheap or a failure to effectively negotiate with vendors.

Failure to carefully plan content. Many organizations are careless about the choice of content and their content provider. The quality and depth of the content are important considerations as site visitors are generally looking for useful information, and they will go to another site if they do not find it here.

Lack of integration with other marketing activities. Many healthcare organizations fail to fully integrate their on-line marketing with other marketing activities and with the organization's strategic plan. Websites are treated as stand-alone information and promotional vehicles that are not well integrated into the other marketing efforts of the organization.

Assuming that the project is finished. As some point, healthcare organizations assume that "it's over." However, it is never "over" when it comes to websites. The Internet is dynamic and involves an evolutionary process that requires constant attention.

Failure to make a long-term commitment. When revenue or volume improves, healthcare organizations often decide to slash marketing budgets. When the organization faces a crisis or downturn, marketing people often get the boot, despite their pivotal role in business development, cost-cutting, and revenue-enhancement strategies. The organization must be prepared to support on-line marketing efforts with on-going management resources and regular maintenance.

Source: Used with permission from Thomas, Richard K. (2007). *Marketing Health Services.* Chicago: Health Administration Press, p. 316.

Box 11.4 The HIPAA challenge to healthcare marketing

The Health Insurance Portability and Accountability Act (HIPAA) of 1996 – presents a challenge for the marketer who must find acceptable ways to take advantage of the data that the organization has access to. Fortunately, the majority of marketing efforts that healthcare providers are involved in are allowable under HIPAA definitions of marketing as are most of the types of communication covered entities conduct with their patients.

One rationale for the acceptance of marketing under HIPAA standards involves the extent to which the relationship between caregiver and patient must be maintained. Within this trust relationship, providers should be able to send information to their patients about recommended screenings and immunizations, new procedures, treatments and health-related seminars. The avowed purpose this activity is to improve wellness, disease management, quality of life and longevity.

Under HIPAA rules, doctors, hospitals, pharmacists and health plans are allowed to communicate freely with patients about individual treatment options and other health-related information, including disease management, case management and care coordination. It is even permissible to disclose a patient's information for marketing purposes assuming that the individual has authorized such disclosure. The use of aggregate data on patients is generally allowed and even purchased lists of patients that include geodemographic information. The critical factor, of course, is the masking of any individual's identity.

The majority of marketing programs healthcare entities are conducting today are *not* prohibited by changes to the HIPAA privacy rule and do not require prior authorization. However, marketers are urged to obtain an opinion from the organization's legal counsel or a HIPAA consultant.

presents a barrier to uses of data that individuals in other industries would take for granted. (Box 11.4 discusses HIPAA issues related to marketing.)

It is likely that such techniques will be slowly but surely incorporated into healthcare, and particularly into those components such as pharmaceutical distribution where there are less qualms about the use of data. The demands of a competitive and consumer-driven system will require it, and contemporary consumers themselves are likely to insist upon ever-more interactive access to healthcare providers.

Chapter 12
Measuring the Effectiveness of Marketing

The importance of measuring the success of a marketing initiative should be a primary consideration, and mechanisms for assessing both the efficiency and effectiveness of a marketing campaign must be built in on the front-end. Measuring the impact of marketing initiatives allows marketers to determine the success of the effort and justify the costs involved. This chapter addresses the uses of evaluation in marketing and presents various techniques that might be applied.

What is Evaluation and Why is it Important?

Evaluation is an essential component of the marketing plan, and its functions include monitoring the progress, measuring the efficiency, and determining the effectiveness of the initiative. Evaluation allows us to answer the questions: Have we met marketing goals and, if so, how efficiently have we done it? The evaluation process provides checks and balances to the initiative, helping to ensure that deadlines are met, budgets are adhered to, and the project otherwise stays on track. The evaluation and feedback phase of the marketing process assesses the effects of the project as a whole as well as the individual elements of the campaign. Evaluation occurs throughout the marketing process, not just at the end, and feedback is used at each stage to improve the initiative.

Ultimately, the marketing effort will need justification, and this requires an adequate evaluation effort. The evaluation process allows for the introduction of midcourse corrections and provides useful insights into the development of the next marketing initiative. The gist of each evaluation effort should be a set of "lessons learned" that can be applied to future initiatives.

Senior management (including marketing management) should care more about the evaluation of marketing campaigns than anyone else. After all, they are the ones who will be judged (and presumably rewarded) based on the effectiveness of the marketing effort. Evaluation should be carried out not only because it is the right thing to do and important for "checking one's work," but also because healthcare administrators are going to be increasingly demanding justification for marketing expenditures.

There are other stakeholders who may have an interest in successful promotional efforts as well. Staff members within the organization clearly have an interest in the impact of promotional activities. Feedback from the evaluation effort provides an appreciation of the type of response that may be anticipated from the public and the expectations customers will bring with them. Members of the organization's board of directors have a clear interest in the quality of the marketing effort, not just for its results but for what it says about the organization.

Funding agencies such as foundations (not-for-profit) or investors (for-profit) have an interest in the effectiveness of marketing from their respective positions. Even government agencies funding a demonstration project or research effort may have a vested interest in how effectively the project was promoted.

Finally, colleagues in both healthcare and marketing are likely to have an interest in the effectiveness of various marketing techniques. Other healthcare organizations may hope to benefit from your experience, and other marketers may consider applying a successful technique in another setting.

Why It's Harder in Healthcare

There are a number of factors that make measuring the effectiveness of marketing more difficult in healthcare than it is in other, more traditional industries. Some of the more significant factors are discussed below.

Goal Issues. The marketing goals of a healthcare organization are often less clearly defined than those of other industries. There is often a diffuseness to their marketing goals, and it is not unusual for different departments of the healthcare organization to have unsynchronized if not incompatible agendas. Special attention, then, must be paid to carefully specifying project goals and assuring that they are realistic and appropriate for a healthcare setting.

Success Issues. In healthcare, the standard criteria for success might not be applied as they are in other industries. Most healthcare organizations do not have the strict bottom-line orientation that other companies have. It may be considered inappropriate to even talk about "profit" within some organizations, and some services may be offered with the expectation that they will never show a profit. Yet, these services may be required by law, may be necessary to counter a competitor, or may be demanded by the public.

Measurement Issues. Perhaps the most important reason that healthcare marketing is different has to do with the various indirect effects that need to be considered. There is seldom a direct link between a service that is provided and the flow of revenue that it produces. An urgent care center may barely break even financially but may steer patients to the health system's physicians and into its inpatient facilities. A marketing campaign implemented for the urgent care center, thus, cannot be evaluated in terms of its contribution to the financial bottom line of the clinic itself but in terms of the indirect impact that it has on the organization and its bottom line.

Diverse Influences. Another consideration in healthcare relates to the variety of factors that influence the use of health services. In other industries, it is often possible to isolate the effect of a marketing campaign because other factors are not likely to come heavily into play. That is not the case in healthcare where a variety of factors may influence customer behavior, including changes in referral patterns, shifts in health plan coverage, and changes in reimbursement patterns among others. These are all variables that the healthcare organization has little control over but are, nonetheless, likely to have a greater impact on patient behavior than any marketing campaign.

Lack of Emphasis. Historically, neither marketers nor administrators have placed much emphasis on the evaluation of marketing initiatives. For marketers, evaluation is usually the least interesting part of the job. Healthcare administrators should be very concerned about the evaluation of marketing campaigns but often show little interest. Needless to say, both marketers and administrators need to get beyond this barrier so the marketing process can be effectively carried out.

Misconceptions About Evaluation

To these barriers one can add the misconceptions that exist that impede the evaluation of marketing in healthcare. A frequent deterrent is the mystique that surrounds evaluation. It is often thought of as some arcane endeavor that requires special skills, equipment and methods. For the most part, evaluation can be carried out with paper and pencil and an observant eye. There need not be anything mysterious about it.

There is also the notion that evaluation requires specially trained experts who can master the mysterious art of evaluation. While many types of evaluation should not be attempted by "amateurs," most evaluation techniques can be easily learned. It may be necessary to engage an evaluation consultant if a lot is at stake. At the very least, a professional evaluator might be used to help set up the methods that are to be used and for analyzing the more technical types of data. Ultimately, this should be an activity that can be mostly carried out in house.

Related to the above is the notion that evaluation is complicated. Like any scientific endeavor, it can be as complicated as we want it to be. But it doesn't have to be very complex. Much of process evaluation involves basic record keeping, and anyone who can read participant rosters, progress reports and schedules can track the progress of the project. Admittedly, the evaluator needs observation skills that might have to be honed, but none of this is rocket science.

"Back end" types of evaluation such as outcome, impact and cost evaluation can be more complicated and may require more complex skills. But, like a lot of things, the better the process that is put in place on the front end, the easier the implementation. Carefully laid out (and measurable) objectives will facilitate the process, and the ability to track results is critical. Again, it may be necessary to bring in an evaluation expert for some aspects of effectiveness assessment and cost analysis, but these are skills that eventually should be brought in house at a large healthcare organization.

Finally, evaluation does not have to be perfect. If it did, nothing would ever get evaluated. There are some things in healthcare that are simply hard to measure (e.g., what actually accounted for the change in admissions or the true return on the marketing investment). Ultimately, we have to measure the aspects of the project we can and not worry too much about the parts we can't measure. Being able to evaluate some aspects of the campaign is better than not evaluating any of it. The perceived barriers to evaluation that exist can usually be easily overcome. Rather than being deterred, it is essential that the healthcare marketer resolves to overcome them.

Types of Evaluation

Once the questions to be answered through the evaluation process have been identified, the next step is to decide which methods will best address those questions. A marketing campaign can – and should – be evaluated in a variety of ways. Multiple methods of evaluation are particularly useful in healthcare, where the intangible benefits of a marketing initiative are often as important as the tangible ones. The major types of evaluation are described below.

Process Evaluation

Process evaluation assesses the efficiency of the marketing initiative by documenting the steps in project implementation and providing feedback on the campaign's progress. The number of factors involved in process evaluation can be considerable, with the factors chosen for evaluation depending on the nature of the campaign.

Process evaluation deals with at least three aspects of the marketing initiative: task completion, role performance and content development. The assessment of task completion involves an examination of the extent to which the appropriate steps in the process were taken in the right order and the various milestones were reached.

The analysis of role performance determines the extent to which appropriate parties participated and how well they fulfilled their roles. For more "academic" evaluations, assessing role performance is a matter of professional competency. For applied settings like healthcare the objective is more practical – i.e., is everyone doing what they need to be doing to get the job done? Ultimately, success depends on the right people in the right positions effectively performing their roles.

In considering the content aspect of process evaluation, the evaluator assesses the consistency of the message and examines the extent to which the same point is made in various contexts. This might examine the extent that clear, unambiguous messages are used to communicate the point of the initiative and assess attributes such as readability, comprehension level and so forth. The main question for the evaluator is: Does the campaign convey the correct message in an appropriate manner?

Some of the methods to be utilized in process evaluation include: a monitoring and feedback system; member surveys about the initiative; goal attainment reports; behavioral surveys; and interviews with key participants.

Process evaluation should also consider the degree of integration of the various components of the marketing initiative. This would determine how well the various aspects fit together to form a coherent campaign. In this respect, the project might be evaluated in terms of the acceptability, compatibility and synergy of methods utilized.

Process evaluation might consider the extent to which the target audience is exposed to the campaign. It would consider the number and timing of print advertisements or television or radio spots. It would measure the extent of distribution of posters, billboards, and other materials.

The implementation plan formulated at the beginning of the project should provide the basis for process evaluation. It will include the list of tasks to be performed, the timelines for task completion, the resources allocated, and the division of labor. Each of these factors can provide the basis for benchmarking. (Box 12.1 presents a checklist for use in process evaluation.)

Box 12.1 Checklist for process evaluation

This checklist can be used as a template for tracking process evaluation activities. The bullets can be filled in with the details of the specific project.

Tasks to be completed:
-
-
-
-

Roles to be performed:
-
-
-
-

Resources to be used:
-
-
-
-

Materials to be produced:
-
-
-
-

Deadlines to be met:
-
-
-
-

Outcome Evaluation

Outcome evaluation focuses on the *effectiveness* of the marketing campaign. It is one thing for tens of millions of viewers to be exposed to a commercial during the Super Bowl. It's another for some portion of those viewers to change their behavior because of the advertisement. Outcome evaluation measures, among other factors, changes in knowledge, attitudes, preferences and behavior. Knowledge may be measured in terms of top-of-mind awareness of the organization, its brand or its services. Attitudes may be measured in terms of the level of positive perceptions of the organization or service being marketed. Preferences can be measured in terms of expressed preference for a particular organization's services. In every case, these are metrics that can be assessed before and after the marketing campaign.

The key measurement areas to track include awareness of the product, advertising awareness and recall, knowledge level, attitudes and perceptions, images of the product held by consumers, experience with the product, and actual consumer behavior. The questions asked about the particular product or campaign should be very specific.

Changes in behavior can be measured at the individual level or at the organizational level. At the individual level this information can be discerned in the same manner as knowledge, attitudes and preferences. The behavior of the target population can be measured via pretests to determine the frequency of use of a particular service or purchase of a particular product. Looked at differently, behavior can be measured in terms of movement from a nonuser status to a user status or from seldom-user to frequent-user status. Measuring the effectiveness of the campaign in this manner requires a considerable amount of research, but the results are worth the effort. (Box 12. 2 presents a checklist for outcome evaluation.)

Box 12.2 Checklist for outcome evaluation

Event participation
Consumer exposures
Column inches
Changes in:

    Volume
    Revenue
    Profit
    Market share

Consumer responses
New customers
Changes in customer satisfaction
Changes in consumer perceptions
Changes in consumer knowledge
Changes in consumer behavior

Box 12.3 Examples of impact measurement
Change in market share
Change in overall perceptions
Changes in consumer lifestyles
Changes in incidence/prevalence rates
Improvement in market positioning

Impact Evaluation

Impact evaluation assesses whether or not the marketing campaign actually induced the desired change (e.g., an increase in consumer approval or greater patient volume). The actual impact of the marketing program is often difficult to assess accurately. Can one public service announcement produced by the health department through its social marketing initiative, for example, cause a drop in morbidity and mortality from heart disease? Probably not, but along with many such efforts combined synergistically it may be a contributing factor to health status improvement. Because marketing campaigns are relatively short lived, it may be difficult to determine the effect of a particular advertisement on overall trends.

An example of the difference between outcome and impact evaluation relates to a social marketing program aimed at HIV-infected individuals. To the extent that the initiative was successful in reducing the amount of risky sexual behavior would be related to outcomes. An actual decrease in the incidence of HIV infection would reflect impact.

Impact evaluation has more relevance for social marketing than for more traditional promotional activities in that community-wide impact is important. A follow-up survey can identify the extent of attitude and behavior change in the target population, and tie it to their exposure to the campaign or use of the product. A "user profile" can be compiled, either from the KAP survey or from additional studies of users and nonusers. Evaluation efforts can also utilize secondary sources to determine changes in behavioral measures. (Box 12.3 presents a checklist for impact evaluation.)

Cost Analysis

Marketers are increasingly asked to justify any marketing initiative in terms of its costs. Cost analysis requires detailed record keeping with regard to both the expenditures and revenues associated with the marketing initiative. Some type of cost–benefit analysis should be conducted prior to the initiation of the project, and every effort made to track the benefits that accrue to the organization as a result of the marketing effort.

The financial benefits associated with an initiative can be measured through either a cost–benefit analysis or a cost-effectiveness analysis. A cost–benefit analysis involves the systematic cataloging of effects as benefits (pros) and costs (cons), valuing those effects in monetary units, and then determining the net benefits of the proposed initiative or activity relative to the status quo. Some cost analysis can take place concurrently with the campaign, but most of it will occur after the campaign has been completed and enough data have been collected to gauge the results of the campaign. (This is another area where it might be worthwhile to obtain input from an outside expert.)

A cost-effectiveness analysis may be used to assess the comparative effects of expenditures on different health interventions. Therefore, defining the core concepts of "effectiveness" is necessary. A very simple definition of effectiveness in health-related activities is that health services are considered effective to the extent that they achieve health improvements in real practice settings. A cost-effectiveness analysis requires a numerical estimate of the magnitude of the effects of an intervention on desired outcomes. This is usually expressed in a cost-effectiveness ratio which is the difference in effectiveness between an intervention and the alternative. A more practical measure might be the cost per unit of outcome (e.g., new customers generated).

Although evaluation techniques are often praised for their bottom-line objectivity, they are also useful in healthcare where it is not possible to place a dollar value on everything. Thus, cost-effectiveness analysis can take into consideration the intangible aspects of the service delivery process. Rigorous cost–benefit analyses are likely to be less suitable for use in healthcare than in most other industries.

Increasingly, health professionals are being asked to justify a marketing initiative in terms of its return on investment (ROI). Some type of financial analysis should be conducted prior to the initiation of the project and every effort made to track the benefits that accrue to the organization (in terms of visibility, perception, market share, volume, and revenue) as a result of the marketing activity. Not only does this task require a carefully constructed marketing plan, but it demands detailed record keeping with regard to both the expenditures and revenues associated with a marketing initiative.

There are a number of factors that make ROI measurement a challenge in health-care, and other measurements (market share, brand position, preference, etc.) are likely to have more validity (and measurability) in the long run than does ROI. These factors include the time delay in the appearance of marketing results and the fact that the use of health services is not likely to be triggered by marketing but will be situational. Further, many efforts toward marketing health services simply don't have a measurable return. Ultimately, we are left with the fact that a variety of factors are likely to influence the use of health services.

A major issue in healthcare is the lack of access to the necessary data – on both the expense and revenue sides. Healthcare organizations typically cannot accurately isolate the costs associated with a marketing initiative from other factors, nor can they precisely determine how much of incremental revenue can be attributed to a marketing initiative. How, for example, can the role of referrals be accounted for, and how does the organization account for revenue generated in other areas besides the targeted service line (e.g., inpatient admissions resulting from an urgent care center campaign)?

Given that most of the ROI measurement assumptions do not hold true in health-care, traditional methods for ROI measurement are not particularly relevant. Health professionals need to determine what factors are meaningful to measure and develop the support systems for measuring them. Marketers should measure ROI for single, specific efforts and/or situations where the measurement systems are relatively good and are up to the challenge. (Box 12.4 addresses the issues of ethical considerations in marketing.)

Box 12.4 Is the marketing initiative ethical?

Marketing initiatives should be subjected to an ethical evaluation – and this is particularly important in healthcare. A number of different concerns have been raised over the years related to claims made for health-related goods and services, the endorsement of various products, and the marketing activities of health professionals and organizations. Ethical criteria must be considered from the beginning in selecting the target audience, designing the research and determining the marketing mix and applied during the evaluation process to make sure the initiative "does no harm." Every element of the program must be ethically sound.

Whenever marketers attempt to influence behavior, it is imperative to acknowledge the need for responsibility and accountability to the people in the target audience, and this a particular consideration when it comes to healthcare. Although in the end, the results of the program are the final measure of success, the means to that end are just as important. People should never be coerced into a behavior, even though it may be "for their own good." Programs that offer incentives for behavior change should be discouraged if behavioral change is not necessarily in the best interest of the customer.

The promotional activities of healthcare organizations should avoid misleading or exaggerated claims and not offer inappropriate incentives for the use of services. Celebrity endorsements should be factual and spokespersons should be able to support the claims that they make on behalf of the organization. The marketer may not have the same perspective as senior management when it comes to decisions on marketing ethics, and every effort should be made to keep everyone on the same page. This is another area in which involvement of the organization's management is likely to be crucial.

Ultimately, however, the ethical principles of the healthcare organization should assure the integrity of the marketing campaign. There is a bond of trust between healthcare providers and their customers, and the dependent relationship that patients have with clinicians makes them particularly vulnerable to misleading claims. All marketing should reflect professionalism and healthcare marketing should place an emphasis on integrity and honesty in advertising. Ultimately, any marketing activity should be an accurate reflection of the organization's mission.

The evaluation process should consider the consequences of marketing activities – both intended and unintended. Indeed, early in the marketing planning process, when objectives are being considered, it is important to hypothesize about the likely consequences of the proposed action. It is usually relatively easy to identify the intended consequences; after all, that is what the process is all about. Identifying the potential unintended consequences requires somewhat more creativity. There have been numerous incidents when carefully planned and expensive marketing blew up in an organization's face because of a failure to consider all of the implications of the initiative.

There are examples of marketing initiatives that have offended large segments of the patient population, alienated certain stakeholder groups, or raised questions about the character of the organization. Marketing initiatives by hospitals have been known to give the impression that they were competing with their medical staff or

---

Box 12.5 The curse of unintended consequences

Perhaps the greatest challenge in evaluating a marketing initiative relates to the identification and measurement of unintended consequences. Speculation on potential unintended consequences should be initiated early in the process, at the time when the goals and objectives are being formulated. For each objective, for example, the potential consequences – both intended and unintended – should be considered. "What if" scenarios can be constructed to prospectively assess the impact of the initiative on existing utilization patterns, the organization's image, referral relationships, and established partnerships.

The perceived benefits of an aggressive marketing initiative should be balanced by the potential backlash on the part of various parties. The benefits accrued, for example, from attracting a few additional customers should be examined relative to the impact on existing customers or on referral relationships.

The following questions might be asked pursuant to assessing potential unintended consequences:

- Who might be turned off by the initiative or any aspect of it (e.g., the tone of an advertisement)?
- Will new competitors be created as a result of the campaign?
- Will a response from existing competitors be provoked?
- Will existing partners feel slighted?
- Will consumers form an undesirable perception of the organization as a result?
- Will the "wrong" kind of customers be attracted?
- If the initiative is successful, can we adequately manage the response?

to prompt a competitor to aggressive action that they might not have otherwise taken. Admittedly, not all consequences of a marketing campaign can be anticipated but the more that can be identified on the front end the better off the organization will be. (Box 12.5 describes some issues related to the unintended consequences of marketing.)

Collecting Evaluation Data

The manner in which evaluation data are collected depends on the nature of the marketing initiative, the promotional technique being utilized, and the type of evaluation that is being carried out. A number of techniques can be used for collecting relevant data.

Record keeping. The most common means of collecting the relevant data for process evaluation is through record-keeping activities. On a very basic level, this would involve keeping track of the meetings that are held (and recording minutes), the level of participation of various parties, the expenditure of funds by the project, and other basic administrative and record-keeping activities. This would also involve measuring the extent to which the participants met the various milestones in the plan and the extent to which prerequisites were in place at the appropriate time.

Observation. The evaluator should have regular interaction with marketing staff and consultants. By observing their activities the evaluator can obtain information on their efficiency and effectiveness. The more systematic the observation the more effective it will be. At the same time, the administration of the healthcare organization should maintain regular contact with the evaluator, thereby observing the actions of the project manager and gauging the progress of the project.

Media tracking. Media tracking involves the measurement of the number of advertising "spots," the number of viewers exposed to a promotion, the number of community meetings held, and other indicators of the activities of the initiative. This is information that should be available as a result of the record keeping inherent in the project.

Surveys. For measuring changes in knowledge and attitudes, it is common to pretest members of the target population with regard to the parameters that the marketer is attempting to influence. This might be accomplished by administering pretests to establish a baseline for knowledge and attitudes, followed by posttests administered to the same or similar respondents. The difference between the pretest and the posttest can be assumed to be a result of the effect of the marketing campaign. These "recognition tests" can be used to determine the extent to which the public has been exposed to a campaign and what type of impression it has made on them.

Experiments. There are also circumstances in which experiments might be used to determine the impact of a promotional campaign. This technique is frequently used in the pretest stage of product development during which members of an experimental

group are exposed to certain information or activity and members of a control group
are not. The changes in the knowledge, attitudes and preferences of the experimental group are presumed to reflect the impact of the "treatment."

Data Extraction. Outcomes can also be measured using data extracted from various
internally maintained databases. The most obvious of these are the information
systems that track patient activity and service provision. Every healthcare organization maintains records on the number of patient visits and admissions. Those with
call centers and customer relationship management systems are likely to track
inquiries and other patient contacts. Organizations keep records of the number of
diagnostic tests provided and the number of treatments performed.

Not only can changes in these metrics be tracked in absolute terms, but it is even
better if they can be tracked in relative terms. For example, if our volume is up 10%
presumably as a result of our marketing campaign, it would be important to determine that our competitor's volume was not up commensurately. If everyone
increased their volumes by 10%, then it's hard to argue that the marketing campaign was responsible.

This same issue can be approached from a market share perspective. If information is available on the total number of procedures performed for a particular procedure, it is possible calculate the organization's market share and then track it over
the time period of the marketing campaign. Thus, if the number of cases of
Procedure X increases by 10% but there is no overall increase in the total number
of procedures performed for the service area, it can probably be assumed that market share has increased as a result of the marketing campaign.

An important aspect of the operation that should be tracked relates to financial
changes that occur. It is common to track the level of sales over time, the revenues
that are generated, and changes in the level of profitability. The organization's
accounting system should be able to provide this information in enough detail to
determine if the targeted service, for example, accounts for the changes in revenues
or profitability. (Box 12.6 presents examples of metrics that might be used for the
evaluation of a marketing initiative.)

Box 12.6 Examples of evaluation metrics

It might be worthwhile to examine some of the indicators that can be utilized to measure the effectiveness of a marketing campaign. The "metric" to be used depends on the nature of the campaign, the promotional technique utilized, and the type of evaluation that is being carried out. Examples are provided below.

Public relations
- Press releases distributed
- Press conferences held
- Articles published
- Media mentions
- Enquiries generated

Community outreach
- Number of community events
- Participation in community events
- Volunteers employed
- Community awareness
- Enquiries/leads generated

Advertising
- Media placements
- Consumer exposures
- Consumer responses
- Ad recall
- Consumer perception
- Consumer awareness
- Increases in volume, revenue, etc.

Direct marketing
- Direct mail pieces distributed
- Outbound calls made
- Inbound calls fielded
- Responses generated
- Leads generated
- Customer conversion rate
- Cost per contact/response/new customer

Sales promotion
- Promotional items distributed
- Literature distributed
- Consumer exposures
- Traffic volume at exhibits
- Leads generated

(continued)

Box 12.6 (continued)

Personal sales
- Sales calls logged
- Leads generated
- Negotiations initiated
- Contracts finalized
- Sales volume
- Cost per sales call/sale

On-line marketing
- Site visibility
- "Hits" to website (overall, pages)
- Visitor response
- Visitor interactions
- Leads generated

Customer relationship marketing
- Size/completeness of consumer database
- Number of inbound calls fielded
- Number of outbound contacts generated
- Customer response
- Customer satisfaction

Chapter 13
How to Be a Healthcare Marketing "Hero"

This final chapter of the book takes a straightforward approach to what marketers can do to make themselves heroes in the eyes of their organization. These ideas go beyond the basics of doing a good job as a marketer to bringing that additional "value added" dimension to the table. Marketers who pursue these objectives will move their organization a long way toward becoming a "marketing organization."

The Effective Healthcare Marketer Should...

Be the expert on the market. In the past, it was not important for health professionels to know very much about the market. Sure, they had to know who their main competitors were and keep tabs on them. But market research is not a familiar activity to most health professionals, and even those with some interest in profiling the market were not likely to have the necessary skills. Today, virtually every decision that has to be made in healthcare should be prefaced by the question: "What are the implications for the market?" The marketer needs to be ready to answer such questions on the fly without a lot of additional research. There's nothing more gratifying than hearing the CEO say: "I can just call Marketing and get that information."

Be the expert on the characteristics of your customers. Just as health professionals had possessed limited knowledge about their market, they've often possessed even less about their customers. In the past, knowing a lot about their customers wasn't all that important. They knew there were plenty of them and reimbursement was essentially guaranteed. The healthcare world has changed and any providers who don't know their customers well are going to be at a serious disadvantage. It's to the point where it's not good enough to know *something* about the customer, but we need to know *everything*. Healthcare executives are not in a position to acquire this knowledge, and they rely on the marketing resource for this function. When someone asks: What's the payor mix of our OB patients?," the marketer should have this information at his or her fingertips.

Be the voice of the organization (i.e., the administration). In a large healthcare organization, it's not unusual for the public relations or communication staff to "speak" for the administration. Indeed, this is part of their job. But the marketer's role goes beyond being the organization's spokesperson vis-à-vis the outside world. In his every action, the marketer should be presenting the perspective of the organization's management. Whether the activity involves a press release, a direct mail campaign, or a television advertisement, it should be as if the CEO were talking. This means it is not just the words of the executive that should be apparent through marketing activities but his philosophy as well.

Provide input into strategic direction. One of the major changes that has occurred as marketing has become more accepted in healthcare has been the increased involvement of marketers in determining the organization's strategic direction. The once-marginalized marketer may actually be "at the table" today in the guise of a vice president or other high-level executive. This means that there is an opportunity to not just react to strategic issues that are raised but to proactively contribute to the organization's strategic direction.

Demonstrate the value of marketing. Despite the growing acceptance of the marketing function within healthcare organizations, there is a need to constantly demonstrate the value of marketing. Like many things, making a convincing case for marketing at some point doesn't mean it is going to stay made. The organization in general and its executives in particular need to be reminded in every way possible of the value that marketing brings to the organization. Some of the areas for which this point can be made include:

> *Increasing the organization's visibility.* Every healthcare organization needs to be highly visible to one or more constituencies, and this responsibility falls primarily to the marketer. Every marketing activity should involve at least some intent to improve visibility. It can be very gratifying for the CEO to be at a nonhospital function and have strangers comment on how visible his organization is.

> *Enhancing the organization's reputation.* As noted at the outset of this book, marketing is all about reputation management and the responsibility for this rests primarily with the marketer. This does not only mean that specific marketing campaigns should focus on reputation enhancement but that every marketing activity – from the development of collateral material to a major advertising campaign should be developed with reputation enhancement in mind. This also means that the marketer must inject a marketing orientation into the DNA of the organization so that every employee *knows* that they are personally responsible for maintaining and improving the organization's reputation.

> *Building the business.* If reputation management is the primary responsibility of marketing, building the business is a close second. The time when marketing didn't make a difference in the financial success of the organization is long past, and marketing efforts are increasingly contributing to increases in patient volume, revenue, profit and market share. The ability of marketing to contribute to the bottom line may be the single most important argument to make for justifying marketing expenditures.

Be visionary/think outside the box. Healthcare executives who are occupied with keeping the operation running and fighting fires are not likely to have much time to be visionary. And the nature of their training is not likely to encourage them to think outside the box. No one is in a better position to see the marketplace's big picture than the marketer, and the market research available to the marketer gives him access to a perspective that healthcare administrators are not likely to have. The creativity that goes into an award-winning marketing campaign can be directed to the marketplace, allowing the marketer to see opportunities that others are not likely to see.

Constantly present new opportunities. Part of being visionary involves being constantly on the alert for new opportunities for the organization. Some opportunities may be identified within the organization, but most of them are to be found in the marketplace. Some areas in which opportunities should be explored include:

> *Target populations.* The marketer should be more attuned to opportunities with various target audiences than anyone else in the organization. These could be opportunities that are presented by virtue of changes in the marketplace – e.g., the aging of the community's population, a new suburb peopled by young families with children, a burgeoning Hispanic population, or a growing youth athletic program generating sports injuries. This should include new ways of looking at existing populations and involve, say, converting OB customers into pediatric customers or helping older adults transition into the "golden years."

> *Expansion of existing programs.* There are likely to be a variety of services offered by a healthcare organization for which the full potential is not being reached. There are likely to be populations that are not reached by existing outreach programs or segments of the community that are not being reached by existing advertising campaigns. There may be groups of potential patients – e.g., school athletic programs or summer youth programs – that the orthopedic surgeons are not covering. If urgent care centers are in place, there will inevitably be areas that are not served by these facilities.

> *New products/services.* The healthcare field is constantly generating new products and services that could be promoted to existing and potential customers. Although some products are explicitly formulated (e.g., a new use for an existing drug), most of these offerings arise spontaneously from clinical research that is carried out in the process of delivering care. Some of the innovations may be suitable for use with existing customers, while others may require some research to identify potential customers for these new services. The marketer is in a better position to do this than anyone else in the organization.

> *New geographic areas.* Health professionals are not likely to think in terms of the spatial distribution of customers in the way that marketers do. Healthcare providers are used to patients showing up at their door and they typically don't know – and often don't care – where they came from. The marketer should constantly monitor where customers are coming from and, perhaps more important, where they are *not* coming from. In most areas, new communities are being developed and existing communities are constantly undergoing demographic change. The marketer should be alert to that new pocket of potential customers that have not yet been tapped into.

Demonstrate marketing return-on-investment. It is typical for marketers to not consider the measurement of the return on the marketing investment until someone questions marketing's cost-effectiveness. The marketer should not wait to be asked about ROI but should be proactively measuring it. This may take a little extra work on the part of the marketer, but it's better for the marketer to be making these determinations than someone else (who may have an ax to grind with the marketing department). If the marketing effort generates a significant return on the investment, so much the better. If it doesn't, it's better to be aware of this and be prepared to respond to any criticisms that might be raised concerning marketing expenditures.

Identify and promote cost-effective options. In marketing as elsewhere there is a tendency to stick with tried-and-true techniques that allow the marketer to operate within his comfort zone. Unfortunately, some of these techniques may be inordinately expensive and unable to demonstrate much in the way of cost-effectiveness. As noted earlier, marketing doesn't have to be expensive, and, if the marketer is creative, there are a variety of low-cost (or even no-cost) options available to an enterprising marketer. Many of these take advantage of contemporary technology and are not only inexpensive but highly effective with certain audiences.

Implement on-going competitive analyses. Healthcare executives are often so involved in what they are doing that they give little thought to what their competitors (and potential competitors) are up to. Even marketers may investigate the activities of competitors on an "as needed" basis. Just as marketing research should be carried out as an on-going activity, the same is true of competitive analyses. The marketer should have his "ear to the ground" anyway and be in a position not only to react to developments in the competitive environment but to *anticipate* them. Marketers should be able to not only identify quantitative changes in the competitive environment but be able to perceive qualitative changes as well (e.g., dissension within a competing medical group).

Emphasize the educational function of marketing. One of the major functions of marketing is to educate – educate the general public, potential consumers and existing customers. Marketing should be the primary source of information within the community on the organization and its services. Even the most hard-hitting advertisement should have an element of education in it. Further, when detractors attempt to demean what they consider the avaricious actions of marketers, the marketer should be prepared to point out the educational aspect of the promotional effort.

Create a marketing organization. The accomplishment on the part of the marketer that is likely to have the greatest ultimate impact is the establishment of the organization as a true "marketing organization." This means that the notion of marketing is incorporated into every aspect of the organization and that marketing principles guide decision making. The marketing implications of any activity should be considered, and all associates should see themselves as marketers for the organization. Associates should be continuously quizzed on ways to provide better customer service, and corporate representatives should keep their ears to the ground to identify challenges or opportunities arising in the marketplace.

While the marketing department or even an outside agency may have much of the responsibility for the development of specific marketing campaigns, the overall marketing thrust should be driven by a core group of individuals representing administration, clinical operations, medical records, information technology, human resources, and research, in addition to marketing staff or consultants. Creating a team in this manner has the dual effect of ensuring an appropriate range of input into the marketing process and keeping all relevant parties informed of marketing strategies and promotional activities.

Finally, the marketer should be in a position to say – no matter what issue comes up – "Marketing can contribute by..." This means that the marketer must take a proactive approach to the situation and anticipate challenges and opportunities. Fortunately, there is virtually no aspect of healthcare in today's environment that does not have implications for marketing and for which marketing cannot make a contribution. The marketing "hero" needs to be able to make this statement and back it up.

Index

Printed in the United States
107412LV00001B/119/A